HOLISTIC HANDBOOK

This book is intended as a reference volume only and is not a medical manual. The information given in this book is designed for educational purposes to help you make informed decisions about your health. It is not intended as a substitute for any treatment that may have been prescribed by your doctor. If you suspect that you have a medical problem, we urge you to seek appropriate medical care.

The mention of specific companies, organizations or authorities in this book does not imply endorsement by the author or publisher nor does mention of specific companies, organizations or authorities imply that they endorse this book, its author or the publisher.

Internet addresses and telephone numbers given in this book are accurate at the time of publishing.

2020 Ganapati Publishing House

ISBN 978-1-7354196-0-2 ebook
ISBN 978-1-7354196-1-9 (pbk.)

Published in the United State of America.

holistichandbook.co

LETTER FROM THE EDITOR

Coming down with a cold or the flu can stop you in your tracks. What if there was a way to shorten the intensity and duration of these illnesses right from the start?

Brian Dempsey, L.Ac., M.S.T.C.M, has written a thoughtful, comprehensive holistic guide to minimize the magnitude of illnesses such as the common cold, flu, coughs, bronchitis and pneumonia, and sinus infections.

In each chapter, Brian provides in-depth instruction on herbal recommendations, including dosages, as well as other holistic treatments such as acupuncture and manual osteopathic medicine that can often be of help.

For readers concerned about COVID-19, Brian has written a special chapter dedicated to the prevention and treatment of this virus.

Brian has based his writing on the latest cutting-edge research to help guide readers to develop an understanding of how to boost the **Immune Response**, restore **Vagal Tone** and the **Gut Microbiome**, and navigate through the **Stress Response** caused by colds and flu.

Brian's attentive and reflective approach to holistic health empowers readers by providing an awareness of how to protect yourself and your family from catching colds or the flu, and how to implement natural, effective treatments, if you do become ill.

Having practiced Acupuncture and Herbal Medicine for almost three decades, Brian has run one of the most successful holistic clinics in America. Brian's interest in colds and flu began in 1991 during an internship in China. It was there that he interned with a doctor who specialized in colds and flu. Since that time, Brian has updated his knowledge using up-to-date research to guide his clinical practice.

Now, Brian is bringing that wealth of knowledge to readers everywhere through this engaging, helpful guide.

CONTENTS

INTRODUCTION

BEGINNINGS

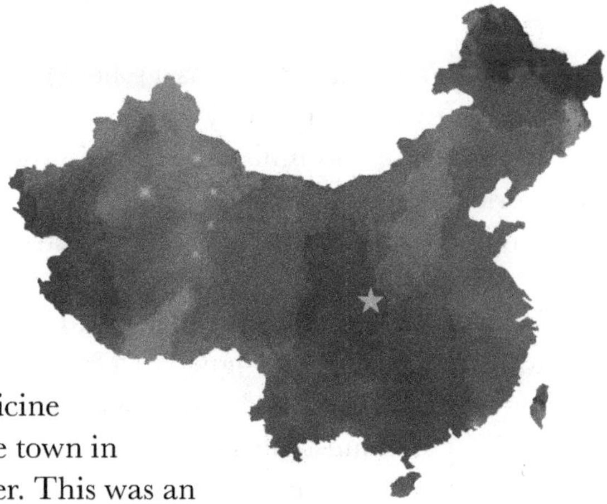

During the summer of 1991, I attended an internship in Chengdu, China at the Chengdu College of Traditional Chinese Medicine. This internship was the final part of my four-year medical degree in Traditional Chinese Medicine (TCM) and I traveled to this remote town in South Central China for the summer. This was an adventure I could never have imagined, when China was still dominated by roads filled with bicycle commuters, street markets, herb shops, and tea houses. While I did have some time to take in the sights and sounds of this vastly different culture, most of my time was spent at the hospital in outpatient clinics where I did my rotations.

Midway through my internship, however, my fellow interns and I had some trials and problems which I never imagined would happen. The situation centered around the Chengdu College administrator, who organized our clinics and classes, and who suddenly informed us that our next scheduled clinic was no longer available. While I did have ongoing conflicts with this person, this sudden cancellation was completely unacceptable as this next clinic was one of the main reasons I had come to China. Our administrator, whom I had nicknamed "the dragon lady," appeared to be pulling a fast one and passing us off to a less-skilled but more politically-connected practitioner. The doctor we had planned on sitting with was a renowned doctor who specialized in the treatment of the common cold and flu.

Coming to China, I was a well-prepared student, having completed nearly 4 years of Chinese medical training at the American College of Traditional Chinese Medicine in San Francisco. However, all of my previous training did not prepare me for the overwhelming experiences of living, studying and attending clinics in China, and this conflict and many other factors made studying in China challenging. For one thing, I had never been in a situation where I lacked basic privileges such as the freedom to come and go as I pleased, or the option to choose the professor I studied with. But this was, after all, the provincial city of Chengdu, in the heart of South Central China, which had, at that time, no interest in bowing to the interests of Western students. Here was a school from a communist nation that had autocratic rules and petty tyrants throughout its government, including, in some cases, administrators within their colleges. It was truly another world. Few spoke English, and people I encountered had little awareness of anything beyond their own life and struggles in their city.

When I arrived in this strange city, I discovered that even if you were going to school, you were assigned to a "work group," complete with work group lodging where you and your group (made up of fellow students) lived along with a communist official who controlled your hours of "work", who you got to study with and most all the other logistics of your life. Our "work group" leader was none other than the dragon lady. Faced with going home unable to study with the doctor that had inspired the trip to China, we fought for the professor we wanted, unsure whether we would be allowed to sit with her. In the end, our temporary standoff ended favorably. She finally relented without even being bribed! I learned in China that stubborn insistence on reaching my goal would pay off, and we were ultimately allowed to sit in with this well-known doctor.

The clinic we gained access to was, like all our other clinics, located in a separate part of the hospital dedicated to doctor's seeing outpatients. Prior to this clinic, we had studied with two other outstanding doctors who were, and remain, husband and wife. Dr. Yang, the husband, essentially ran a TCM clinic dedicated to treating Hepatitis. At that time, Hepatitis A had infected approximately 10% of China's population, and a great number of these very sick patients went to Chinese doctors to receive herbal prescriptions.

After this clinic, we spent another period of time with Dr. Yang, his wife, in a gynecological clinic. Both clinics were fascinating, and the scope and depth of their knowledge were far beyond any of my expectations. However, it was not until we were finally admitted to this next clinic that the most important part of my internship came to fruition. This was the famous Dr. He, who we had so fervently fought to sit in with. I did not know until later that Dr. He was given the nickname "Dr. Gan Mao" by hospital staff. This translates as Dr. Cold and Flu.

When we first arrived at Dr. He's clinic, like the two previous doctors we had seen, there were patients standing in long lines outside her offices waiting to be seen. We arrived in the morning, and as Dr. He started seeing patients, our interpreter relayed all that the patient and Dr. He were saying. Within a few days of observing, I began to realize that I was sitting before a diagnostic master with true skill in prescribing Chinese herbs for patients with colds or flus. In fact, it was reported to me that virtually all the doctors and staff of that hospital came to see her for quick resolution to their colds.

We sat with Dr. He for a little over two weeks, and saw her with almost 40 patients per day. It was disorienting for me to watch her work, as she saw and diagnosed many symptoms that I missed. I still remember when she would turn to me and ask what my diagnosis and prescription was after a patient had stated their symptoms. I can say that, for the first time in my clinical experience in China or America, I had no idea how to diagnose or prescribe at her level. In fact, the only thing I had the good sense to do was to take copious notes, knowing that I would have to spend a lot of time studying them. I knew that if I organized and studied my notes, I could perhaps begin to understand how she was diagnosing her cases and which herbal formulas she was using.

Upon returning to the States, I decided to put all this information into a database to sort it out and then, using this information in a more organized format, slowly reassembled my understanding of treating the common cold and flu in line with the methods of Dr. He. This was an effective way to understand her diagnostic skill and perception so much so that, within a year of my return, I decided to begin writing this book. That was a long time ago, and it is only now, almost 30 years later, that I am satisfied that I have captured the spirit of those Chinese clinics along with the insights that I have gathered from my own clinic experience.

ADOPTING AN INTEGRATIVE MEDICINE APPROACH

A final piece of my background occured later in my career, this time in California. I was invited to be part of a team that taught alternative medicine at a medical school and became a founding member of an Integrative Health Center, participating in regular grand rounds to help doctors find the appropriate alternative therapy to support their patients. These experiences aided me in understanding TCM in light of Western medicine and other healing traditions, and helped me to learn how to put more emphasis on research on herbal medicine and acupuncture. Both were invaluable as they taught me how to look at TCM through a Western, science-based lens and helped me broaden my understanding of how to do in-depth research into the medicine that I had been trained in.

Now, so many years later, I am writing this as a tribute to my teachers, patients and wonderful researchers who have given me knowledge enough to spawn deeper insights into health concerns like the common cold. No one has written an in-depth book for the general public which outlines in detail the elegant and effective strategies set forth using an integrative approach using herbal medicine, acupuncture and other holistic remedies for treating the common cold or flu. Nor has there been a comprehensive effort to bridge these Eastern methods to Western medical concepts about the cold and flu.

My intention is to set forth a scientifically-based explanation and protocols in understandable language. As you will find, this book provides groundbreaking ideas backed up extensively with cutting-edge scientific concepts. Included in this book you will find useful information on hygiene, cold and flu viruses, and the **Immune System** all geared to empower you and your family to take action when faced with a cold or flu. Also included are chapters on stress, sinus infections, coughs, bronchitis and pneumonia with practical measures you can take to speed the healing of these illnesses.

My approach provides a cutting-edge understanding of what I call an **ENS viral cold** or **Flu**, **Low Vagal Tone**, the **Gut Microbiome**, the **Gut Brain Axis** and the **Autonomic Nervous System**. With this modern knowledge base, you will be well armed in combating any cold or flu symptom. The last chapter is for those who seek advice about COVID-19. It will give you concrete steps that you can take to prevent catching this virus. Moreover, it will help you to find herbal medicine that can speed the healing of this scary virus and help you quickly restore the health of you or your family.

CHAPTER 1
Hijacked: Our System is Being Hijacked by a Virus

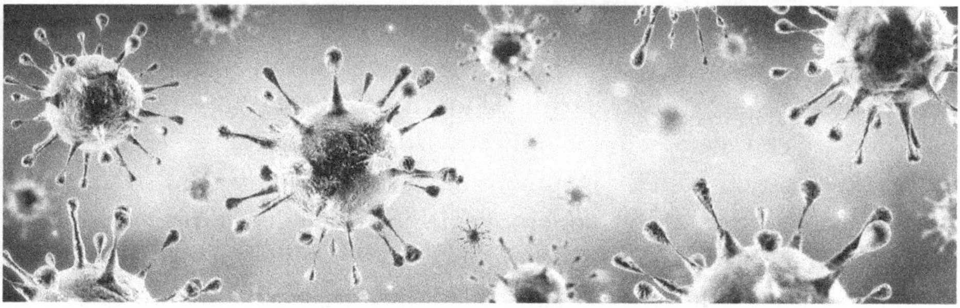

THE VIRUS: A MODERN UNDERSTANDING OF WHAT CAUSES COLDS AND FLUS

This chapter reviews cause and treatment of a cold; we should explore the modern, Western understanding of what causes colds and flu. There's a lot of misconceptions regarding our current understanding of what causes a cold. Many think colds and flu are caused by cold weather or germs. There is also a widely held assumption that antibiotics are a suitable treatment for ridding our system of these germs. In this chapter, I will talk primarily about the chief cause of the common cold and flu: a virus. This understanding will help you better understand not only why Western treatments are ineffective but also why herbal therapies can offer a viable and helpful alternative.

Colds are Primarily Caused by Viruses

The vast majority of colds begin and end as a viral infection. A recent scientific study analyzed whether colds and flu are caused by viruses or bacteria and concluded that "[b]acterial infections [are] rare, supporting the concept that the common cold is almost exclusively a viral disease."[1]

Many are surprised to find that there are over 200 viruses that can cause a cold, and a few that are associated with the flu. In addition, this list of 200 viruses is slowly growing as every few years, a new viral strain appears. The most common cold virus is called the **Rhinovirus**, which is responsible for 20% to 80% of colds each year. The flu, on the other hand, is associated with just a few viruses. These strains are called **Influenza A**, **Influenza B**, and **Influenza C**. Flu viruses tend to be more virulent and create more dramatic symptoms, including high fever or chills and more extreme fatigue and body aches.

There are no accepted Western medical treatments for any virus that causes a cold; there is only palliative care. As for the flu, flu vaccines and patient isolation are considered our most effective strategies. However, these vaccines offer no protection from the common cold and target only a few strains of the flu. To understand why modern medicine, which discovered the cause of colds and flus, but has no cure, we must take a closer look at viruses. Viruses are unique pathogens that are unlike any other, to which our **Immune System** is exposed.

What is a Virus?

A virus is a microorganism, far smaller than bacteria, that is often described as a fragment of a living thing. Each virus particle is known as a virion and is composed of a set of genes (either RNA or DNA) wrapped in a protective protein shell. Viruses are not only smaller than bacteria and other organisms, but scientists can't agree if viruses are living organisms or not. Out of the seven criteria used to determine if something is alive, viruses only pass two of them. This odd fact indicates that finding a drug that "kills" viruses might be challenging. After all, it may be difficult to kill something that isn't a living thing.

Another unique characteristic of a virus is the way they infect us. Unlike bacteria, that simply reproduce by splitting into two identical cells, viruses attach to one of our cells and then enter into that cell and take over the cell and it's reproductive function. In a way, a virus is more like a microscopic parasite that must invade a living cell to reproduce. When a virus successfully invades a cell, it can, by using the cell division mechanisms of the cell, start replicating itself and, in this way, grow into a severe infection. Because they enter into our cells, they can remain hidden from our **Immune Response**, at least for a few days. In the **Immune System** chapter, we will learn the fascinating way that the **Immune System** overcomes this problem.

What is a Novel Virus?

A novel virus is a new viral strain such as the COVID-19 or the SARS-CoV-2 Coronaviruses. Because these viruses are new to humans, our **Immune System** memory cells, which store information on all the infections we have had and help us to combat a virus more quickly, do not have any memory of these viruses. That means these viruses have not only tended to spread more rapidly but have a more extended recovery period. It also means that our **Immune System** does not have memory cells which "remember" this virus, and so the **Immune Response** will be slower. We'll find out more about memory cells in the *Chapter 3: Meeting the Challenge of the Clone Wars.*

How Do We Catch a Cold?

Even though there are a little over 200 types of cold and flu viruses, each type has many strains. For example, the virus called COVID-19, the current pandemic virus, as well as the SARS-CoV-2 virus, which was a novel pandemic virus in 2003, are two subtypes of the same Coronavirus. Each strain of cold or flu virus, including **Rhinovirus**, can have many subtypes. Viruses are typically transmitted by a person or animal that is already infected who sneezes or coughs. This is the primary way that viruses are transmitted.

The most common way of becoming infected is through breathing the air that has virus particles embedded in droplets. Breathing the air contaminated with virus particles is especially problematic in a closed environment like an elevator or airplane where one or more persons that have a cold, sneezes or coughs. For a few minutes after some sneezes, the air can remain saturated with the cold virus. Keep in mind that not everyone that sneezes has a cold.

These airborne viruses are also deposited on surfaces around them and passed to others when we breathe the air or touch the surface that has viral material and then touch our mouth, nose, or eyes. The membranes of the eyes, nose, and mouth are porous enough to allow the virus to pass into our bloodstream and begin its parasitic mission. Even an open wound can serve as a staging area for viruses to enter into our bodies. Cold and flu viruses are more likely to be found in public spaces with heavy traffic and a low cleaning regimen. An infected person can spread their virus with a sneeze or cough which is then passed along to others.

When one or more viruses enter into your system, you will likely "catch" this cold. Viruses must enter our bloodstream and attached to a cell to begin replicating. Within hours of this happening, most people will start exhibiting typical symptoms such as a sore throat, fatigue, and sinus congestion.

How a Virus Infects Our Cells

All viruses replicate in our bodies by attaching themselves to a cell and hijacking the cell's inner workings. Through the injection of a virus's genetic material, the virus is able to take over the cell's replication, reproducing many more viruses into the system. The whole process is called the Lytic Cycle and explains how viruses hijack many of our cells and replicate exponentially. When the virus population expands to a certain level, we experience the symptoms of a cold.

Once a virus begins to replicate, it can quickly create a whole army of identical virally-infected cells. This exponential replication is the beginning of what will turn into the clone wars between the virus and certain parts of our **Immune System**. I will review this phenomenon in *Chapter 3, Meeting the Challenge of the Clone Wars.* Suffice to say, few other pathogens can infect us so quickly and expand so dramatically.

What Affects the Viability of Viruses?

How long a virus can survive once it's deposited on a surface depends on many factors. Below are some of these factors.

1. **HUMIDITY** – Humidity is less conducive to viral viability. In a CDC study, higher humidity resulted in a significant reduction in a virus's ability to infect.
2. **COLD WEATHER** – A recent study by Dr. Zimmerberg, an NIH scientist, found that the protective outer membrane of viruses held up better in cold weather (slightly above freezing) and did far worse in warm weather (60°F and above).

3. **TYPE OF VIRUS** – **Rhinovirus** does not survive more than an hour when deposited on surfaces, but the Coronavirus such as the SARS-CoV-2, the virus from the 2003 epidemic, could survive up to 3 days on metal and plastic. This same Coronavirus was found to be able to survive for several hours in the air.
4. **TYPE OF SURFACE** – In general, viruses survive longer on hard surfaces such as stainless steel and hard plastic, and not as long on softer surfaces such as fabric or cardboard.
5. **TIME** – Viruses usually only remain viable for a few hours, at most, after being deposited on a surface.

On a practical level, this list could help us make wiser choices when protecting ourselves and our family from catching a cold. We should be more vigilant with prevention in cold weather. Also, we should avoid contact with hard surfaces such as handrails, doorknobs, or elevator buttons in public spaces, or at least wash our hands or use hand sanitizers after touching these kinds of surfaces. In certain circumstances, such as an airplane, we reduce the risk of being exposed to viruses by wiping down all the surfaces with disinfecting wipes.

What is the Difference Between a Viral Cold and a Bacterial Cold?

Viruses are tiny infectious particles approximately 100 times smaller than bacteria. Bacteria are much larger, single-cell organisms. Viruses don't have all the inner workings of a bacterium and, unlike bacteria, cannot reproduce on their own. Bacteria also create an infection by multiplying in the extracellular fluid and producing toxins that cause inflammation. By contrast, viruses enter the extracellular fluid as a staging area to find and enter into a cell where it then hijacks the cell's reproductive function. In terms of treatment, bacteria can be treated with antibiotics, but viral infections are not treated directly with any medication.

A bacterial cold is a rare thing. It is possible, however, to catch a secondary bacterial infection such as bacterial pneumonia or a sinus infection that may require antibiotic treatment. This is why doctors now often refrain from prescribing antibiotics when their patients report that they have caught a cold or flu.

Hygiene Practices

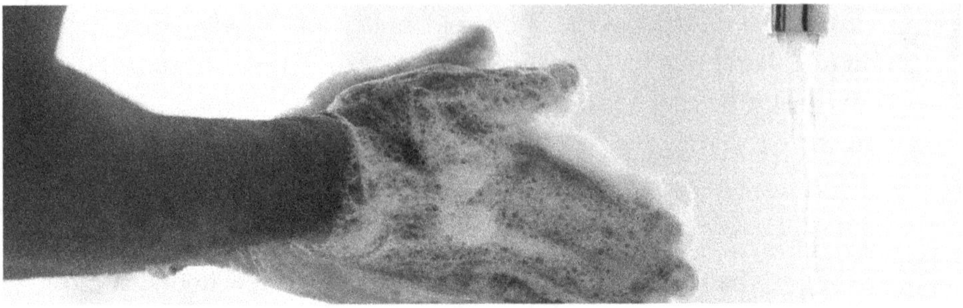

Hand Washing

The most important and effective thing you and your family can do to prevent catching a cold or flu virus is to wash your hands. The CDC says you should wash for at least 20 seconds with soap and warm water. The temperature of the water is important in order to disrupt the lipid coating of the virus.

Face Washing

Technically, the reason the CDC places so much emphasis on hand washing is so that you don't touch your germ-laden hand to your face. My suggestion is to also wash your face with warm water. This is why wearing gloves doesn't make sense as you could pick up a virus on your glove, then touch your face, just the same as with a bare hand. The great news is that simple warm water and soap can eliminate viruses that you may have unknowingly picked up by touching a contaminated surface.

Isolation, Quarantine, and Social Distancing

All three of these practices are recommended to prevent the spread of a virus. Isolation and/or quarantine means that if you catch a cold or flu, you should isolate yourself from everyone. If someone helps you, make sure that they are wearing a mask and thoroughly washing their hands and face after seeing you. Social distancing is a practice where everyone in a community stays at home to avoid contact with an infected person. Social distancing is an extreme measure that is only utilized during a pandemic, such as the COVID-19 Coronavirus.

Clean, Clean, Clean

When you or a family member has a virus, you should clean everything they touch, at least until their sore throat or fever has completely abated. That means cleaning their pillow cases, door knobs that they have touched, their phone, their dishes, and anything else that they use. If a sick family member has traveled in your car, clean the space that they occupied, including door handles and seat belts. If you are in a public space, such as a train station or airport, you should use hand sanitizer to clean your hands after touching surfaces. When on an airplane, bus or train, you should use disinfecting wipes to clean tray tables, armrests and all the surfaces around you. In an elevator, try not to touch anything and, if you push a button, clean the finger you used when you get to your desired floor.

What To Do if Someone Sneezes or Coughs Next to You

If someone sneezes or coughs close by, leave the space as soon as you can. Try to hold your breath and immediately go to the bathroom and wash your face and hands. If you have no choice, then cover your face or turn away when this happens.

Avoid Crowded Places

Crowded places present more risks of catching a cold. Avoid when possible.

Masks

Masks are a controversial method of protection, at least in the United States. The CDC now recommends healthcare workers use them and that the general public also use some kind of face covering for pandemic flus. In Asia, masks are already considered to be almost mandatory when going out. More evidence is now emerging that masks can help prevent the spread of a virus. I agree and am in favor of wearing a mask during a pandemic when in public or at home if you are sick and your family is not.

Hand Sanitizers

Hand sanitizers should be used when warm water and soap are not available. The most effective hand sanitizers have at least 60% isopropyl alcohol content. If store-bought hand sanitizers are not available, rubbing alcohol (90% alcohol) with some aloe vera can be a good alternative. An example of a homemade formulation is shown below:

- ⅔ cup of 90% rubbing alcohol
- ⅓ cup of aloe vera gel

This mixture can also be sprayed onto contaminated surfaces and wiped vigorously to eliminate most pathogens.

How Long are People Contagious?

While there are exceptions to the rule (like the Coronavirus Covid-19), patients who catch a cold are usually only contagious for two to three days from the start of exhibiting symptoms. Five percent of those tested were still contagious after 2.9 days. The fact that the patient is contagious for the first three days provides a compelling argument for isolating your family members when they first come down with a cold or flu. It is also important to frequently wash clothing, pillowcases, and eating utensils of the patient to lower the risk of infecting others.

What Distance is Safe to Keep From an Infected Person?

A 2011 study concluded that viruses can infect people within six feet around them after coughing or sneezing. This six-foot spacing also applies to more contagious viruses such as the Coronavirus COVID-19.[2]

How to Eliminate a Viral Infection with Alternative Medicine

Surprisingly, killing off these marginally alive fragments of existence is difficult. To my knowledge, killing off only the virus within a virally-infected cell is almost impossible. For one thing, when a virus inhabits another cell and takes over its functions, it is virtually impossible to extract the offending virus from the cell, nevermind finding a way to kill it. If there are no drugs or herbs, and our **Immune System** cannot kill a virus, then how do we get rid of these virulent parasites?

The answer is a bit shocking. To kill off the virus, we must kill the cell that it occupies. So as we engage in our herbal quest to eliminate a viral infection, we must also kill millions of its cloned cells, which used to be healthy cells. The main therapeutic focus of this book is to help stimulate the **Immune Response** to help our **Immune System** to kill infected cells. There is a very detailed description of this process and how to do it in *Chapter 3, Meeting the Challenge of the Clone Wars.*

Of course, in the process of killing off the virus and the cell it occupies, the body must withstand the assault and death of millions of its cells while remaking new cells to replace the diseased ones. This process of killing off and remaking cells alone can help explain why recovering from colds and flus is so tiring and requires so much rest. As we will learn in *Chapter 3, Meeting the Challenge of the Clone Wars,* gearing up and subsequent suppressing of the **Immune Response** also draws a lot of energy.

Inhibiting Viral Infections

There is another approach to fighting off a viral infection that scientists have explored employing drugs that inhibit viral replication. All antiviral drugs currently on the market work by inhibiting virus replication. Although the drugs that have been approved by the FDA have shown some promise, scientists have found that many viral strains are demonstrating **Resistance** to these drugs. Readers should keep in mind that none of these drugs are currently part of the standard of care for colds or flus.

Although it appears some herbs can inhibit a virus from replicating, my experience with this line of treatment is less consistent than that of using medicinal herbs to help our **Immune System** eliminate virally-infected cells. I do, however, find one herb promising in inhibiting viral replication. This herb is called Schinus Molle (Brazillian Peppertree) and it is the most common herb used in South America for the treatment of the common cold and flu. Preliminary research on Schinus Molle demonstrates that this promising herb inhibits viral replication.[3,4] I have, at times, used an alcohol percolation of this herb topically to some benefit. Although it is not the main focus of this book, I do rely on this herb with specific patients and hope that the scientific world will put more attention on the therapeutic properties that it appears to possess. More information can be found about this strategy and how it works at the end of *Chapter 4, The Body's Secret Regulator.*

I recently found out through colleagues that TCM herbal medicine was used extensively during the Wuhan outbreak of the COVID-19 virus. They stated that many Chinese people during the height of the COVID-19 pandemic utilized a TCM formulation called Qing Fang Bai Du Tang. This TCM formula purportedly inhibits virus replication; however, I don't think that scientists have rigorously investigated this claim. I am hopeful that science will soon turn its attention to these and other herbal formulas.

A Virus Only Dominates the First Phase of a Cold

The viral infection within our system leads to symptoms that include a sore throat, fever, and fatigue. At some point, all these symptoms diminish and other symptoms appear, such as a cough, a sinus infection, or bronchitis. This second set of symptoms is what I call the second phase of a cold. In the second phase, the viral infection has mostly been defeated, and the remaining symptoms appear as a result of the **Immune Response**'s attempt to clean up the debris from the battle between the **Immune System** and the virus.

As I walk you through all aspects of a cold, you will finally feel empowered to take action to help yourself and your family successfully treat colds and flu.

Can a Virus Infect the Enteric Nervous System?

One of the central premises of this book is that colds and cases of the flu, no matter which strain, are usually an infection of the **Enteric Nervous System** (**ENS**). The **ENS** is a vast network of nerves located in the gut and sometimes referred to as the **Second Brain**. This assertion is backed up by years of my own clinical experience, and validated by many recent scientific studies. The idea that cold and flu viruses primarily attack nerve tissue is not unheard of. For instance, Shingles or Bell's Palsy are viral nerve infections that demonstrate how viruses can infect parts of the nervous system.

As you read through the next few chapters, you will find much of what I have discovered is grounded in cutting-edge research that explores new medical concepts that are changing the landscape of modern medicine. Concepts such as the **Gut-Brain Axis**, **Low Vagal Tone**, and the **ENS** are fundamentally the new landscape of healthcare and will change many of the premises of modern medical practice. In the next chapter, we will begin to explore this fascinating new understanding of the common cold and flu.

CHAPTER 2
The Second Brain: Target of the Cold and Flu Virus

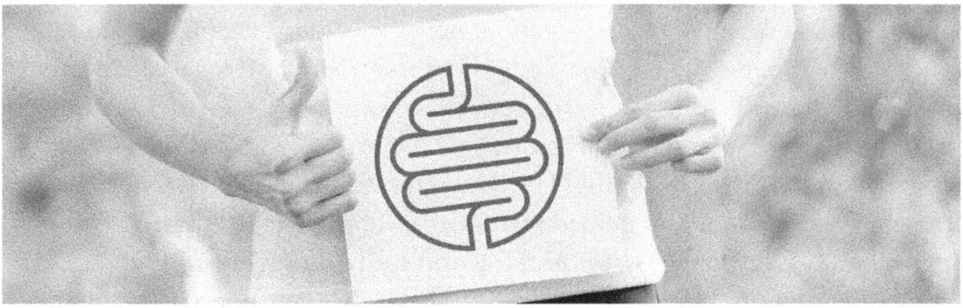

The **Second Brain** is a relatively newly discovered brain that resides in our gut. When I became aware of this new part of our anatomy, I was intrigued and started to work with it using acupuncture and later using herbs. The **Second Brain** is called the **Enteric Nervous System (ENS)**, and although dedicated scientists are devoting their careers to uncovering the secrets of this hidden brain, few therapies have yet been discovered that work with it. As an acupuncturist, I decided to begin to work with my patients using acupuncture points that correspond with this area, and surprisingly, I found that it was a key to understanding and treating the common cold and flu. In this chapter, I will talk about a patient, who is actually a composite of many patients, to describe my process of discovery. The revelation I had, after many years of work, was that the **ENS** was directly related to colds and flu.

Around 2005, I saw a patient whom I'll call Mary. Mary is the patient that helped me to unravel some of the mysteries of the **Second Brain**. Mary comes to see me from time to time for a variety of complaints. During one such occasion, Mary asked me to try to alleviate some of the discomfort she was feeling from her cold. It turned out that Mary had the type of head cold that I see most frequently at my clinic. She came in with a sore throat, a stopped up nose, low-grade fever and chills, and the beginning of the fatigue that accompanies most colds.

THE SECOND BRAIN COLD AND FLU: A NEW UNDERSTANDING

Of course, physicians would diagnose this presentation of a cold as an upper-respiratory infection. A **TCM** (Traditional Chinese Medicine) diagnosis would be a "Wind-Heat Cold." More information is available about this and other **TCM** diagnoses in Appendix A. As I was already exploring alternative treatments, I deviated from the standard **TCM** diagnosis and tried something new. This chapter is about the evolution of my thinking that led to this new approach. More importantly, it's about how my understanding has shifted and radically changed my approach to the treatment of colds and cases of flu. As you will come to understand, incorporating the **Second Brain** into the diagnostic differential is a radical departure from **TCM** as well as conventional medical thinking. However, this non-standard way of treating the common cold and flu helped my patient Mary far more than anything that I had used before. As my thinking and study progressed, I found a surprising amount of research which validated this new approach.

SYMPTOMS OF A SECOND BRAIN (ENS) COLD

To properly introduce the innovative strategies of this chapter, I must first give you a few more of Mary's symptoms, symptoms to which she was unaware until I pointed them out. Below is a more complete list of Mary's symptoms:

- Sore throat.
- Fatigue.
- A very stiff neck, particularly the back of the neck, verified by palpating on the upper part of the back of the neck (C-1 through C-3 zone). Mary immediately confirmed the tension that I felt.
- A tight knot in the muscles at the top of the stomach, just below the sternum. Pressing down in this area, the knotted muscles were touch-sensitive.
- A feeling of heat in the upper abdomen; heat as in a low-grade fever. Confirmed by using an infrared thermometer on this area. The temperature corresponding to her stomach was 96, while the rest of her body read 87 degrees.
- Sinus congestion.
- A mild headache. Headaches associated with colds are usually centered in the forehead or over the eyes, although, for some patients, it can be a headache over the left or right temples. Less than one quarter of the patients that I see have a headache as part of their cold, but it is common enough to mention here.

As a stiff neck was prominent in Mary's case, I diagnosed this as a **Tai Yang/Stiff Neck cold**. (See Appendix A for more details on this diagnosis.) While evaluating and treating a stiff neck associated with a headache was something I did frequently, a stiff neck accompanying a cold or flu was something that seemed unrelated to the cold or flu. Nevertheless, the **TCM** diagnosis of this cold, and many others I worked with, was this mysterious **Tai Yang/Stiff Neck cold**. This problem is compounded by the fact that **Tai Yang/Stiff Neck cold**s, as most **TCM** diagnoses, are based on symptom patterns rather than on the modern biomedical model.

A TAI YANG/STIFF NECK COLD

As I worked in an integrative health consortium that included medical doctors, it made me a bit uncomfortable adopting a diagnosis that was difficult to explain to my colleagues. During this timeframe, however, I was able to start to unravel this mysterious diagnosis in a way that began to make sense. Before I put the pieces of the puzzle together, let me remind the reader just how seemingly disjointed the symptoms of a **Tai Yang/Stiff Neck cold** are. A **Tai Yang/Stiff Neck cold** may include these symptoms:

- A stiff neck.
- Sore throat.
- Chills and fever.
- Sinus congestion.
- Fatigue.

While a stiff neck is a central feature of the **Tai Yang/Stiff Neck cold** pattern, yet I had trouble relating this musculoskeletal problem to a viral cold or flu. Moreover, it was difficult to connect the stiff neck to other cold symptoms such as sinus congestion, sore throat, or fever.

Before this, I rarely ever asked about a stiff neck when a patient presented with a cold and, consequently, a **Tai Yang/Stiff Neck cold** was a diagnosis that I rarely thought about. Furthermore, patients rarely report a stiff neck, even if they were aware of it, as they were more focused on symptoms such as their sore throat or fatigue. At the time I saw Mary, because I had many patients who complained of stiff necks and headaches accompanying their cold, I began treating these patients using the **Tai Yang/Stiff Neck cold** diagnosis more frequently.

As I became more familiar with this diagnosis, I began to routinely check patients for a stiff neck when they reported having any cold symptoms. The results of this change in my routine resulted in a surprising outcome, as I found almost everyone I checked who reported having a cold also had a stiff neck.

Even with this change, however, the **TCM** treatment for **Tai Yang/Stiff Neck cold** was somewhat lacking. The herbs and acupuncture treatment that I had learned in China only helped a bit. Patients reported that while their symptoms were somewhat improved, the duration of the cold appeared to be only modestly improved. Nevertheless, this small breakthrough of connecting a stiff neck to colds and flus left me questioning my whole approach to treating colds and flu, and left me wondering if there was a more effective treatment of these illnesses.

EPIGASTRIC PAIN: A NEW DISCOVERY

As I continued to work with patients in this new way, I discovered another significant insight into **Tai Yang/Stiff Neck cold**s. During this time, I began to notice the connection with **Tai Yang/Stiff Neck cold**s and the area below the rib cage, which is just above the stomach, called the **epigastric area**. Strangely, this area seemed to be somehow related to having a stiff neck. I frequently noticed a pronounced feeling of heat and tension as I palpated over this area when a patient reported cold or flu symptoms. Abdominal heat and tension was so common that I began to think of this heat as a low-grade abdominal fever. With this new insight, the next time I saw Mary for a cold, I found this new understanding to be quite helpful in relieving her symptoms. I decided to insert acupuncture needles in the **epigastric area** and with this new treatment, Mary reported that her neck relaxed and her sore throat began to go away within minutes of inserting the needles.

Around this same time, I also discovered a book written by Michael Gershon, M.D., who teaches at Columbia Medical School. The name of the book was *The Second Brain*, and because of the groundbreaking information which it contained, I began to rethink the **Tai Yang/Stiff Neck cold**. Gershon's book began to explain the connection between the **epigastric area** and the neck. The main premise being that a separate nervous system, embedded within the abdominal muscles surrounding the stomach and intestines, has a remarkable influence on our health. He dubbed this separate nervous system, the **Second Brain**, which scientists call the **Enteric Nervous System** (**ENS**).

THE SECOND BRAIN CHANGES HOW TO LOOK AT MANY HEALTH PROBLEMS

Before I discuss the connection of the **ENS** to the neck, I should talk a bit about the unique collection of nerves in the gut and how they function. The first unexpected discovery that Dr. Gerson made about the **Second Brain** (**ENS**) is that it has qualities similar to that which science attributes to the brain. Thus the name "**Second Brain**." The **ENS** is capable of directing action within the body, such as the complex activities of digestion. Unexpectedly, Dr. Gerson also found that the **ENS** can operate independently from our central brain (**CNS**). This revolutionary finding of Dr. Gerson's work on the **Second Brain** extensively documents the "executive" brain-like function of this network of nerves. While the headline around his work was the discovery of the executive brain-like functions of the **ENS**, Dr. Gerson also found that our two brains are highly connected, and there is a great deal of communication happening between them. As we will find in the *Chapter 4, The Body's Secret Regulator*, this communication is related not only to the process of digestion but also integrally involved in the **Stress Response**. Refer to the information box for more information about Dr. Gershon and the **ENS**.

It is this communication between the two brains that captured my attention as I tried to make sense of the connection between the **ENS** and the neck. This connection is called the **Vagus Nerve**, and I have discovered a treasure trove of information about it. Before I get into the details about this set of nerves, I need to point out that the **Vagus Nerve** pathway travels from the brain (**CNS**) through the back of the neck to the chest and the abdomen as well as the **ENS**. This solidified my quest to understand colds and flus on a different level, and kept me studying for several years to fully understand the connection between the gut, neck and the brain.

As my understanding of the common cold was transformed by reading about Dr. Gerson's discoveries, providing a new lens with which I could understand the common cold and flu, I also began to explore research on Viral Tissue Tropism, the study of how tissues support cold or flu viral proliferation. An example of this is a study written about the H5N1 flu virus found in Influenza. A viral replication was present in the intestines and lungs.[9] Other studies have found that viral replication can take place in the gastrointestinal organs as well as the lungs.[6,7] All this added fuel to the fire, as I began to relate colds and flus to the gastrointestinal organs and by association, the **ENS**.

The Second Brain

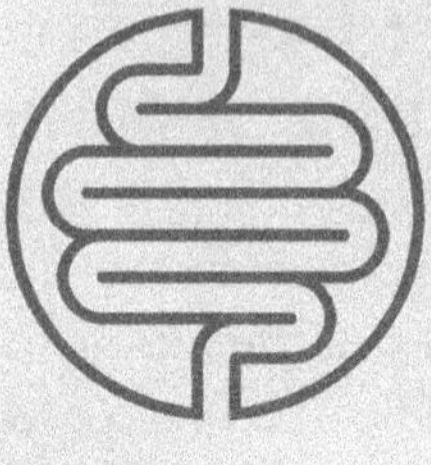

The **Second Brain**, technically called **Enteric Nervous System (ENS)**, is a relative newcomer in the medical world, first championed by Dr. Gershon. This brilliant doctor serves as a professor at Columbia University and has written numerous scientific papers on the **ENS**, and as well as a book on what he calls "The **Second Brain**." Dr. Gershon discovered that this little-studied set of millions of neurons are embedded in the entire abdomen cavity providing a second intelligence in the body. His first discovery was that, among other things, the **Second Brain** drives the digestion processes such as peristalsis and the release of digestive enzymes.[8]

Dr. Gershon discovered the **ENS** during his study of quadriplegics, many of whom had relatively normal digestive function despite the fact that they had severe spinal cord injuries. Dr. Gershon speculated, and later proved through s cientific studies, that there was an alternative system of nerves that provided direct input to all the digestive processes as well as communication between the brain and the gut. His work led him to identify a large nerve network in the stomach that was previously unstudied. The name of this network is the **Enteric Nervous System** or **ENS**.

Through his many years of studying it, he found that:

1. The **ENS** is a brain, meaning that it could control the digestive processes without significant input from the first brain or Central Nervous System (CNS).
2. The **ENS** could complete basic tasks such as shutting down the digestive process when the body is under stress.
3. It connected to the brain stem through a pair of nerves collectively called the **Vagus Nerve**.

As Dr. Gershon continued to study the **ENS** in more depth, he made another startling discovery. The **ENS** not only helps to direct the digestion process but also produces neurochemicals such as **Serotonin**, **Dopamine**, and **GABA**, along with scores of other chemicals that strongly affect mood and energy.[5] The startling thing about this discovery is that prior to this discovery, doctors believed that neurochemicals in the brain were exclusively produced in the brain. Dr. Gershon continues to explore this fertile field, exploring the intersection of neuroscience, gastroenterology, psychiatry and immunology. Since this discovery, Dr. Gershon has garnered attention around the world and is leading a caudry of talented scientists to continue to investigate the **ENS**, the **Gut Microbiome** and the neurochemicals produced. Gershon received the Henry Gray/Lippincott Williams Wilkins Scientific Achievement Award in 2000, and was chosen as a fellow of the American Association for the Advancement of Science in 2007 in recognition of his outstanding work.

Before we return to Mary and her treatment, let me go over the details of the **ENS**. Here I want to highlight how reading Dr. Gershon's book helped me to understand **Tai Yang/Stiff Neck cold**s and transformed my understanding of common colds and flu.

Connecting the ENS to Viral Cold and Flus

Dr. Gershon's groundbreaking work with the **ENS** is a game-changing discovery in the medical world that may have far-reaching implications. In my case, it helped me to identify the **ENS** as an integral part of the viral infection that creates a cold or flu. As I saw more and more patients with the common cold that year, I began to palpate and take temperature readings of this **ENS epigastric area**. I noticed that frequently, tension and heat in the **Second Brain** zone consistently correlated with their cold.

Since nearly all the patients with tension and heat in the **ENS** area also had a tight neck, I began to speculate that these two phenomena were related. So much so that I noted that if the neck was stiff, it was likely that the **Second Brain** area was tight and inflamed, and if the **Second Brain** area was inflamed or tense, it was very likely that the neck would be stiff.

NEW BEGINNINGS: CREATING A NEW TREATMENT FOR ENS VIRAL COLDS

This high correlation between the neck and **ENS** area prompted me to begin to incorporate acupuncture in the **ENS** area as part of my treatment for nearly all of my patients seeking treatment for the common cold, even if they did not report any symptoms related to the neck or abdomen. My new treatment protocol yielded remarkable results with patients. Performing acupuncture in the **ENS** area tended to both loosen the neck and reduce the low-grade fever in the abdominal area. More importantly, patients reported dramatic temporary relief from their cold or flu symptoms. As a result, I became more and more intrigued by **ENS** treatments with acupuncture for colds and flus as well as many for other conditions that involved neck tension, including headaches and stress.

Beyond these remarkable results, I also found that patients that had this treatment, reported that they felt less stressed and more optimistic after an acupuncture treatment. Because the **ENS** produces 95% of the body's **Serotonin** and half of the **Dopamine,** I also speculated that a viral **ENS cold** could affect one's mood and motivation. I quickly found this to be documented research.[10,11,12]

With all these new insights, I began to expand the clinical picture of a common cold or flu. These included:

1. A tight neck, particularly in the back of the neck; especially the first and second cervical vertebrae and the corresponding muscles along the neck.
2. A warm or feverish area just below the rib cage where a significant part of the **ENS** resides.
3. A sore throat.
4. Sinus congestion.
5. Low energy that accompanied a feeling of being sick.
6. Low mood, either depressed or anxiety.

With this new understanding and treatment, I hypothesized that the typical common cold could be a viral infection of the **ENS.** Gershon's book had, at least for me, successfully turned conventional wisdom on its head for the common cold and flu. As you read on, you might find that you will have to reboot your basic understanding of what a cold or flu is, and how it affects the body. To help with this, I will now review the details of how a viral **ENS** infection causes a neurological chain reaction that creates many symptoms.

How a Cold Virus Infecting the ENS Can Cause Cold Symptoms

When the **ENS** becomes infected with a virus, it creates a fairly typical cold or flu constellation of symptoms. I will explain how this chain reaction creates these symptoms due to an inflamed **ENS** in the next two sections. Before we review this in detail, let us look at the **ENS** in more depth so we can understand how important it is to our sense of health and well-being and how, when inflamed, it can significantly alter our health.

SECOND BRAIN AND THE STOMACH

The **ENS** is embedded within the entire abdominal cavity; however, I find that the symptoms of inflammation tend to reside in the upper abdomen, just below the rib cage. This area more or less overlays the organ that occupies this zone, the stomach, and is called the **epigastric area**. It might not be surprising then, that as the **ENS** becomes inflamed, the stomach also tends to become inflamed.

Naturally, the more inflamed the **ENS** is, the more inflamed the stomach will become. As the stomach becomes inflamed, generally the area of inflammation is concentrated at the junction between the stomach and the esophagus. At the junction, there is a valve which is called the **Lower Esophageal Sphincter**. This is an area that can, when inflamed, lead to significant symptoms. The name generally given to these symptoms is reflux or **GERD**. The full medical name for this is **Gastroesophageal Reflux Disease** but most people know it as heartburn. There is also a milder version of **GERD** that is associated with the **Stomach/Lower Esophageal Valve** inflammation. This milder version is called **Silent Reflux**.

SILENT REFLUX IS THE CAUSE OF OUR SORE THROATS

Silent Reflux is a newly discovered medical condition which is, in effect, a more subtle version of **GERD**. The typical reason that people have **GERD** or **Silent Reflux** is the same: either an ulcer or a hiatal hernia. The reason **Silent Reflux** is gaining attention is that the symptoms generated by this milder version of **GERD** can be very detrimental to one's health. Yet, they are often subtle and, so, often go unnoticed. Beyond this problem, there is a wide variation of symptoms that **Silent Reflux** can cause, and these symptoms appear, on the surface, to have little to do with the stomach. Below I have provided a complete list of symptoms associated with this condition:

- Trouble swallowing.
- Sore throat.
- Pressure or mild burning in the chest.
- Itchiness in the upper pallet or ears.
- A sense of fullness in the upper abdomen.

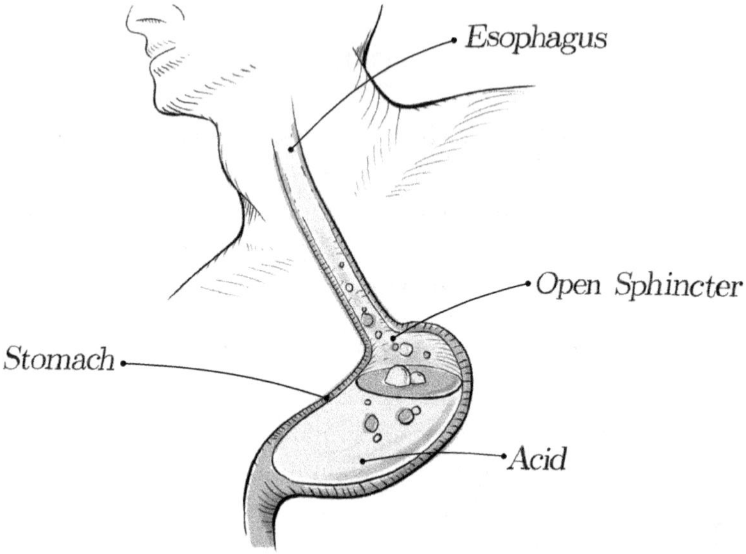

To explain this non-intuitive connection between the stomach and the throat, chest, and upper palate, we need to look at what is happening. When the stomach becomes inflamed, it always means that it and the surrounding tissues have become swollen. Because the **ENS** overlies the stomach and diaphragm, this inflammation causes swelling, not only in the **ENS** but also, in the organs and structures just below it. The Stomach and the **Lower Esophageal Valve**, which is embedded in the diaphragm, also become swollen. The swelling in and around this valve can easily cause the valve to become "leaky," causing a small upsurge of acid to travel up the esophagus to the throat.

Unlike typical **GERD** symptoms, which leave little doubt that you have a medical problem, the symptoms of **Silent Reflux** may only present as a mild sore throat on waking, trouble swallowing, or a sense of stuffiness or tension in the chest. With **Silent Reflux**, there are no obvious stomach symptoms like stomach pain or stomach burning.

Now consider the idea that rather than a small stomach ulcer or some other problem usually ascribed as a cause of **GERD** or **Silent Reflux**, that instead, this area becomes inflamed due to a cold or flu virus infecting the **ENS**. Imagine that the inflammation generated by a cold or flu could trigger **Temporary Silent Reflux** symptoms.

Looking at the symptoms of a common cold or flu from this perspective, we can now imagine that if you have an **ENS viral cold** infection, the symptoms would be virtually identical to those found with **Silent Reflux**.

The symptoms include a low-grade fever over the **ENS Zone** and a sore throat, or pressure in the chest, trouble swallowing or a sensation of itching in the throat. All of these symptoms are considered typical common cold symptoms. I am not alone in my hypothesis around this connection as research has already begun to look in this direction.[13,14]

As I became convinced that the common cold was more of an **ENS** problem than a problem with the lungs or an upper respiratory infection, I began treating every patient I saw as an **ENS viral cold** or flu. I would confirm this suspicion, over the next few years, as I treated many patients with colds and noticed my treatments became dramatically more successful.

ENS COLDS CAUSE TENSION IN THE NECK BECAUSE OF THE VAGUS NERVE

We must look beyond the typical **Silent Reflux** symptoms to understand an **ENS cold**. In addition to upper abdominal fever, the most common symptom is a tight neck, especially along the cervical spine in the back of the neck. To understand the mechanism that causes the tension, we need to look at the connection of the **ENS** to the brain. The connection is called the **Vagus Nerve**. This unique cranial nerve travels from the brain stem into the back of the neck, to the chest, and finally, to the **ENS**. All other cranial nerves travel from the brainstem through the neck to the face. Based on the groundbreaking work of Dr. Gershon, we now know that the **Vagus Nerve** creates a dynamic connection between and the Brain (**CNS**) with the **Second Brain** (**ENS**).

The connection of the **Vagus Nerve** can be compromised when the **ENS** is inflamed. The chain reaction caused by an **ENS** viral infection not only causes inflammation of the stomach creating **Silent Reflux**, but also a corresponding inflammation of the nerves in the vicinity. This inflammation compromises the nerve conduction of the **Vagus Nerve**, shunting off and preventing any neurochemicals from traveling up this nerve. The chemical called **Acetylcholine**, normally keeps muscles surrounding this nerve relaxed.[15,16,17]

When I first discovered this biochemical connection, I called this phenomenon the "**Acetylcholine shunt**," which suggests that the inflamed nerve does not deliver sufficient amounts of this chemical to maintain relaxed muscles. Since the **Vagus Nerve** travels up through the **ENS**, into the chest and then into the back of the neck, all of these areas will naturally feel stiff, and the muscles remain tight until the inflammation subsides. I learned that others have been studying this and other phenomena associated with the compromised delivery of **Acetylcholine**; I found a treasure trove of scientific papers that called this problem **Low Vagal Tone**. Much more information on **Low Vagal Tone** will be provided in upcoming chapters.

With this understanding, I could now comprehend how a patient with an **ENS viral cold** or **flu** could have a stiff neck and why some patients could even experience a tension headache. I found that a stiff neck is a defining feature of this kind of cold, and anyone with skill in massage or manual therapy can detect it in a matter of seconds, even if their patient is unaware of it. When I say this is a defining feature, it means that it is always present, again, even if a patient may not be aware until a practitioner palpates their neck.

SINUS CONGESTION, THE TRIGEMINAL NERVE, AND AN ENS COLD

Sinus congestion frequently accompanies colds, and I began to connect the dots on this problem as well. I found that the **Acetylcholine shunt** that is created by a stiff neck is also involved in sinus congestion. As the neck tightens, it causes enough tension to compress other cranial nerves that exit at the junction between the top of the neck and the skull. This final piece of the puzzle also takes a bit of explaining and some knowledge of anatomy to understand fully. The primary cranial nerve being compressed is called the **Trigeminal Nerve**. The **Trigeminal Nerve** exits the side of the upper neck and travels through the jaw, under the ear, then splits into three branches.

The middle and upper branch of the **Trigeminal Nerve** travels in and around the sinuses. Just as inflammation of the **ENS** can cause the neck to tighten, inflammation and tension in the neck can cause the same shunting off of **Acetylcholine** to the muscles surrounding the **Trigeminal Nerve**. Because of this, the muscles over the nasal sinus area tighten, resulting in the constriction of the sinuses. This, in turn, restricts the capacity to breathe freely. If the upper branch of the **Trigeminal Nerve** is affected, it can lead to a headache and should be considered a trigger even if the headache is in the temple or on one side of the head.

To summarize, we see that an **ENS viral cold** or flu infection causes a sore throat (due to **Silent Reflux**), a tight neck (due to poor transmission of **Acetylcholine** to the **Vagus Nerve**), and sinus congestion (due poor nerve transmission to the **Trigeminal Nerve** being compressed at the top of the neck). Let us look at one final symptom, which is common in both the common cold and flu.

ENS INFLAMMATION AND FATIGUE

A last typical cold or flu symptom is fatigue. How many doctors recommend bed rest for cold or flu? Of course, we know that isolating a patient is important so that they don't infect others, but there is also the stark reality that a patient is simply achy and tired from having a cold. There are many reasons why patients become tired from a cold. For one thing, as we will learn in *Chapter 3, Meeting the Challenge of the Clone Wars*, the **Immune System** is generating millions of cells, fighting off the viral infection and, during this process, also killing off thousands of the body's own virally-infected cells. But there is another equally compelling reason why an **ENS cold** virus causes fatigue. To understand this we need to understand the stresses that this infection creates in the body.

Setting aside the impact of ramping up of the **Immune Response**, we can also consider an **ENS viral infection**'s interference with normal digestion. After all, **Silent Reflux** compromises the digestive process. The stomach plays a key role in digesting fats and proteins, and inflammation interferes with this process. I call this phenomenon **compromised nutritional absorption**. Combine this with blocked sinuses (which inhibit the free flow of the breath), along with a low-grade fever (which often interferes with sleep) and a tight neck, and you have a miserable person who is exhausted.

A more compelling understanding of why patients report fatigue has to do with **Low Vagal Tone**. Understanding **Low Vagal Tone** is key to understanding how stress is involved in every aspect of the common cold or flu. I will save this explanation for *Chapter 4, The Body's Secret Regulator.*

PUTTING THE PIECES TOGETHER

So with this background, let us examine Mary's symptoms again. She had:

- A sore throat.
- A tight neck.
- Sinus congestion.
- Fatigue.
- Abdominal tension and inflammation.

It should now be apparent that this is a typical **ENS cold**. When seeing patients like Mary, I often give them a longer treatment, as they can be miserable, exhausted, and stressed. Utilizing acupuncture and herbs provides a straightforward method to lower the **ENS** inflammation.[18,19,20] This safe and natural treatment loosens their necks, helps lessen their sinus congestion, and reduces the soreness of their throats.

The last section of this chapter outlines treatment options and cutting-edge strategies to speed the healing of this cold.

TREATMENT OF AN ENS (SECOND BRAIN) COLD OR FLU

Understanding the underlying cause of the common cold has gone a long way to helping me identify appropriate natural treatments. In the last ten years, I have identified many helpful herbal and acupuncture treatments for both the acupuncturists treating patients with colds in their clinics as well as home care measures. Below, I will go over treatment protocols that patients can show their acupuncturists first, and then I will go over home care options. The herbal treatments shown below can be administered at home or in a clinical setting and, in my experience, are vital to providing a sustained, lasting effect.

ACUPUNCTURE TREATMENT FOR AN ENS VIRAL COLD OR FLU

Acupuncture treatment can be administered at any stage of a cold or flu and will have a dramatic effect on temporarily lessening symptoms and helping the body recruit and deliver more blood flow and immune cells to the **ENS** area. The treatments should be administered only by a licensed acupuncturist qualified to insert the needles safely and effectively. The treatment length should be at least 30 minutes.

The points used are based on that symptoms are present. I have organized the points according to symptom below:

SORE THROAT WITH A STIFF NECK	SORE THROAT WITH CHILLS OR FEVER	SINUS CONGESTION WITH A SORE THROAT	SORE THROAT WITH FATIGUE
Stomach 21,22	Stomach 21,22	Stomach 21,22	Stomach 21,22
Ren 14, 15	Ren 14, 15	Ren 14, 15	Ren 14, 15
Small Intestine 3	Large Intestine 11	Gall Bladder 40	UB 40
Urinary Bladder 64		Cup Gall Bladder 20 for at least 30 seconds per side	
		Cranio-Sacral manual therapy at the anterior superior border of the atlas bilaterally	
		Cup at the TMJ joint if the joint is not properly aligned	

HERBAL TREATMENT OF AN ENS (SECOND BRAIN) COLD OR FLU

For the most effective herbal treatment of an **ENS cold**, please refer to the treatment guidelines in *Chapter 3, Meeting the Challenge of the Clone Wars* along with treatment for **Low Vagal Tone** outlined in the Stress and the Common Cold and Cough and Sinus Infection chapters. I provide an abbreviated list here for reference.

1. To reduce **ENS** inflammation and inhibit the virus replication, take Schinus Molle (Peppertree) applied topically to the **ENS/epigastric area**, especially just below the rib cage.

2. Boost the **Immune System** by taking Reishi, Shitake, Maitake, Chaga mushrooms according to the instructions given at the end of *Chapter 3, Meeting the Challenge of the Clone Wars.*

3. Reduce stomach inflammation from **Silent Reflux**, especially once the fever and sore throat have subsided, with herbs such as Slippery Elm, Marshmallow Root, and/or German Chamomile. Dosing with all herbs should be 300 to 500 mg per dose for an adult. Slippery Elm can also be taken as a tea utilizing it as a powder. As a tea, put a tablespoon in hot water and drink quickly, as this herb will solidify into a gel if it sits for a few minutes. To increase **Vagal Tone**, take herbal bitters. Refer to *Chapter 5, Eliminating Your Cough by Clearing Out Clutter* and *Chapter 7, Let the Acetylcholine Flow* for more information on frequency and dosages.

CHAPTER 3
Meeting the Challenge of the Clone Wars: A Targeted Approaches to Boosting Your Immune Response

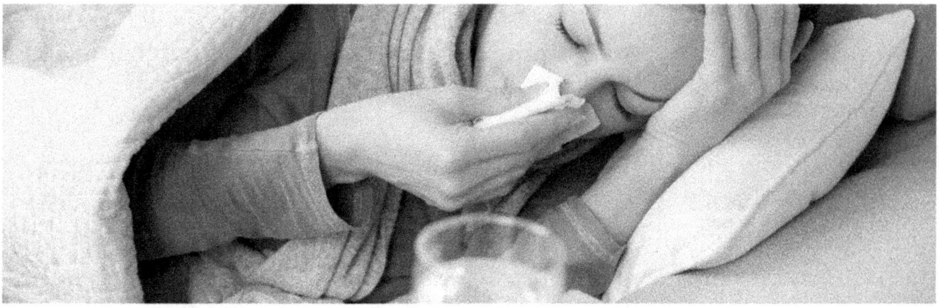

The usual doctor's recommendation for treating the common cold or flu is to rest, drink fluids and isolate. Why? It seems that these benign suggestions were born out of the 18th century when Weir Mitchell, M.D. formulated his book entitled *Rest-Cure.*[21] Fluids came later into the treatment regimen, but even this time-honored piece of advice has been recently discredited.[22] In fact, neither measures seem to help with anything other than keeping a person isolated so they don't infect others. One might rightfully ask why are the mainstream, therapeutic interventions for something as prolific as the common cold limited to 18th-century therapies? The reality is that, after giving modern science more than a century to figure out a cure, there is still no conventionally-accepted treatment for the common cold other than these inadequate or discredited recommendations.

In fact, the medical world seems to have abandoned its efforts to find a cure, and appears to write colds and flu off as "self-limiting," which means they will eventually resolve with no medicine or medical intervention. Implied in this hands-off approach is the knowledge that our own **Immune System** will eventually kick out the offending virus. Given this reliance on our own internal healing system, it can be helpful to learn about it and discover ways to naturally stimulate the **Immune System** and thereby speed the healing process.

IMMUNE SYSTEM OVERVIEW

The **Immune System** is fairly complex and includes many systems within the body that protect us from infection and also help mount a defense to combat an infection or injury. In this chapter, we will explore the **Immune System** and how to support it as a means of preventing colds and flu. We will also look at ways to boost the **Immune Response** as a means of fighting off a viral infection.

Learning about the **Immune System** can be a daunting task as it is fairly complex. To simplify the process, I have compared the **Immune Response** to an army. Specifically, I will compare the **Immune System** to a medieval fortress army, complete with a fortress wall, sentries, combat soldiers, and spies. For, like an army that protects a fortress, the **Immune System** stands guard over us, protecting us from countless bacteria, viruses, and other pathogens. Without it, we simply could not survive this germy world. Also, like an army, there are many different protectors and fighters that each plays a specific role in **ENS**uring our protection.

This cellular defense system can be parsed into many different categories, but in this chapter we will focus on the parts that have the biggest impact on fighting off a common cold or flu. We will first talk about the **Innate** (or non-specific) **Immune Response**. Then we will learn about the **Acquired Immune Response** (specific), which includes the **Humoral** and **Cell-Mediated Immune Response**. Finally, I will discuss the main health issues that suppress the **Immune Response**, and how we can work to reactivate and enhance our **Immune Response** through herbal medicine and acupuncture.

Using our army analogy, we could say that there are several armies that comprise the **Immune Response**. They are typically divided into three categories:

1. **Innate Immune Response**.
2. **Humoral Immune Response**.
3. **Cellular Immune Response**.

At the conclusion of the discussion, I will add a fourth category, the **Natural Killer Cells**.

INNATE IMMUNE RESPONSE

Innate or **Nonspecific Immune Response** is the **Immune Response**'s part of our first line of attack on viruses and other invaders. We say it is non-specific because it performs the same action regardless of the pathogen. We call all invaders **antigens** or pathogens. The hallmark of the **Innate Immune Response** is fever and inflammation which can be seen as a generic, nonspecific response by the body to rid itself of pathogens. Using our army analogy, this could be characterized as sentries that patrol the perimeter marching back and forth to handle relatively minor invasions. The **Innate Immune Response** is a critically important part of the **Immune System**, as it can successfully fight off a minor attack of pathogens and, more importantly, as we will see below, it raises the alarm for other parts of the **Immune System**.

This generic **Immune Response** deploys four main strategies to eliminate pathogens:

1. Generates fever.
2. Creates inflammation.
3. Generates swelling.
4. Releases chemical signals to alert other parts of the **Immune System**.

To look more deeply into the **Innate Immune Response**, we should examine two of its most prominent cells: **Macrophages** and **Dendritic cells**. These **Innate Immune Cells** are classified as phagocytic cells that literally engulf pathogens and thereby kill them. The process of engulfing a pathogen with these cells releases chemicals that, in turn, activate inflammation, fever and swelling. While this is an amazing ability, when you catch a cold, the cold virus gradually enters into our cells, literally hijacks their inner reproductive systems, which enables them to produce billions of replicas of themselves, effectively overwhelming the **Innate Immune Cells**. Nevertheless, these cells, along with the skin and the mucosal lining in the sinuses, mouth and GI tract, serve as a cellular, as well as a physical, barrier to pathogens and helps to delay the onset of a cold.

Everyone is born with an **Innate Immune Response** and so, even babies, who initially only have access to the **Innate Immune Response**, can mount an attack against pathogens. However, anyone who has witnessed an infant getting sick, can attest to the scary process. An infant will typically generate high fevers, become glassy-eyed, lethargic, and sometimes, because of these high fevers, can suffer from intense pain or fever-induced seizures. In this way, infants provide a window into how the **Immune System** functions when only this basic defense system is online. For fever, swelling and inflammation are limited weapons, which are not the most efficient way for the body to fight off a cold virus.

Fortunately, as infants grow up, another part of the **Immune System**, the **Acquired Immune Response**, begins to mature, and as it slowly comes online, the **Acquired Immune Response** helps the **Immune Response** become more balanced and helps fight off colds and flus in a much more effective way.

The Limitation of the Innate Immune Response

It is important to understand that the **Innate Immune Response** has real limitations when it comes to protecting us from catching colds and flus. Obviously, high fevers and lethargy are significant problems, but besides these there are other, less obvious but equally important limitations that you should be aware of. Let's look at the three main limitations:

1. The **Innate Immune Response** cannot "adapt" its response according to which pathogen it encounters, but instead releases the same generic array of chemicals that generate the same kind of fever and inflammation regardless of what pathogen is attacking.
2. Its response cannot change or evolve. This is because the **Innate Immune System** has none of the more specialized **Immune Cells** such as "helper cells" or "memory cells," so it cannot store information about pathogens and over time change to better respond to them.
3. It is concentrated in certain locations in our bodies such as the lymph glands, organs and blood. Because of this, its surveillance and ability to fight pathogens is limited.
4. The **Innate Immune Response** cells, such as **Macrophages**, cannot exponentially increase its numbers as significantly as other parts of the **Immune System**.

Innate Immune Response's Most Important Function

Given these limitations, it can be easy to underestimate the importance of the **Innate Immune Response**. For example, one of their most important functions is to engulf a pathogen, then break it down and display fragments of what the pathogen is (or was) on its surface. This process can serve as a beacon for other parts of the **Immune System**, which serves to sound the alarm and help the rest of the **Immune System** to gear up for a battle. In order to learn more about this beacon, we must learn another term called the **Major Histocompatibility Complex** or **MHC**.

MHCs are fragments of the virus that **Macrophages** and other **Immune Cells** display on their cell surface. As we will see in the next section, these **MHC**s provide a way that other parts of the **Immune System** can "see" and react to viruses, which is critically important to generating a powerful **Immune Response**. We will explore these **MHC** displays in the next section in much more detail so that you can understand just how critically important the displaying of **MHC** is.

ACQUIRED IMMUNE RESPONSE

The **Acquired Immune Response** is the part of the **Immune System** that we acquire as we grow up. The **Acquired Immune Response** is a far more sophisticated and complex system that has an exponentially more targeted response to pathogens. The **Acquired Immune Response** has several unique features that distinguish it from the **Innate Immune Response**, such as its ability to create a **Clone Army** as well as its ability to create and store Memory cells. Below, we will look into some of the intricacies of this system in more depth and see how the **Acquired Immune Response** helps us to fight and conquer a viral infection.

The Two Parts of the Acquired Immune Response

The **Acquired Immune Response** is composed of two separate systems with different cells that work with each system. These two systems are called:

1. **Adaptive Humoral Response**.
2. **Cell-Mediated Response**.

As we will see, these systems share some of the same characteristics, but also have some important unique distinctions between them.

Adaptive Humoral Response

The **Adaptive Humoral Response** is the predominant part of the **Immune System** that dominates the "humors" (an old medical term that refers to the interstitial fluids between the cells). The cell that provides the **Adaptive Humoral Response** is called the **B-cell**, and as we will see, this **B-cell** performs multiple functions within our metaphorical army.

I have divided these functions into three categories:

1. Work as an Army Janitor (much the same way that **Macrophages** work).
2. Create a beacon that alerts other parts of the **Acquired Immune System** leading to the creation of a **Clone Army.**
3. Create specialized librarian cells called **Memory Cells.**

Janitor Soldier Army

B-cells, which are the only cell in the **Humoral Immune Response**, provide several key functions for the **Immune Response**. One of the most important is what I call the Army Janitor function. The **B-cells**, with the help of **MHC**s, helps to find and clean out pathogens from our system.

To explain this in more depth, let us revisit the **Macrophages** from the **Innate Immune System. Macrophages** and other **Innate Immune Cells** find and consume a pathogen like a virus, then engulf the pathogen and display fragments of it on its surface. These fragments are called **Major Histomine Complex** or **MHC**s and make it possible for the **B-cell** janitor soldiers to find and bind with these invaders in the "humors" or interstitial fluids. But, unlike **Macrophages**, only one unique **B-cell**, out of the millions in our system, can bind to the **MHC** displayed on a cell.

Like a janitor with a key ring with billions of keys on the ring, the **B-cells** must find the perfect match of its surface receptor with that of the pathogen in order to eliminate it. The reason these surface receptors can be compared to a key is, like a unique key to a lock, only one of them can perfectly fit and bind to the pathogen or virus, which is necessary in order to eliminate it. Because of this process, it can often take days for the matching **B-cell** to find its match. Once this finally happens, the janitor soldier's job is essentially fulfilled and the next **B-cell** function becomes activated.

Once the Army Janitor **B-cell** finds its match, that matching **B-cell** also displays an **MHC** of the pathogen on its surface and sends out a beacon for another cell called the **T-helper cell**. What happens next is quite amazing, as this is how the process of a **Clone Army** begins.

The Clone Army

Once a **B-cell** finally matches up with a virus, it can, with the help of **T-helper cells**, rapidly expand into a **Clone Army** of identical **B-cells** that perfectly replicate the **MHC**s of the matching janitor **B-cell**. The **Clone Army** can be created in a matter of hours and, once it's created, it quickly binds and destroys the pathogen by the millions and can quell an infection in a matter of hours.

This ability to scale up making millions or even billions of matching clone cells makes the **Humoral Immune Response** exponentially more powerful than any of the **Innate Immune Cells**. However, without **Macrophages** and other cells displaying **MHC**, the **B-cells** can't perform their astounding function at all. The final function of the **B-cells** is what I call the **Librarian Army**. The scientific name is simply **B-Memory cells**.

The Librarian Army

The **B-cell Librarian Army** is exclusively composed of **B-Memory cells**, which carry a chemical "memory" of the matching janitor **B-cell** that was the original **B-cell** cloned and responsible for quelling the infection. This subset of **B-cells** are created at the same time that the **Clone Army** are created so that the next time the same virus strain shows up, the **B-cells** can "remember" the matching **B-cell** and thereby create the **Clone Army** more quickly. As there are many varieties of viruses, we must acquire a "memory" of each variety, as each type comes with different surface receptors.

These **Memory B-cells** help us to adapt and evolve our **Immune Response** over our lifetime so that we can quickly and effectively fight off more and more viruses as we grow older.

B-cell Cloning

When the **B-cell Membrane-Bound Antibody** matches up with a virus, it forms clones of itself creating a **Clone Army** of identical **B-cells** which carry the exact same antibody configuration. When this happens, a special **T-cell** called **T-helper cell** (which we will talk about in the next section) triggers the production of billions of free-floating antibodies that target and eliminate the viral invasion. It turns out that viruses and other pathogens also create Clone Armies of themselves, so this rapid proliferation of cloned **B-cells** serves as an effective counter-attack to the corresponding release of cloned viruses. This counter-attack is a necessary measure that helps our system fight back and eventually win the battle much more efficiently and quickly than with only an **Innate Immune Response**.

The fact that billions of **B-cells** are being matched, cloned and dispatched through the humors, finding and eliminating a rapidly expanding viral infection is daunting. So much intelligent sorting, matching and cloning, along with storing targeted information, gives clues as to just how much energy and resources the **Immune System** uses. It's little wonder that someone fighting off a cold or flu is quite often tired, needing more rest as much of the body's reserves are being used to mount this massive complex defense against a tiny invader. However, the story is not over with the **Humoral Immune Response**, for, as we will soon find, the viruses have a unique ability to hide from this **B-cell** attack, and other parts of the **Immune Response** must kick in to fully eliminate the virus and its clones. But before we look at this, we should examine the benefits and shortcomings of the **Humoral Immune Response**.

The Benefits and Shortcomings of the Humoral Immune Response

Clearly our **B-cell** army is quite versatile and agile in its ability to scout, find and generate a potent **Immune Response** to a cold or flu virus. In the process, it also catalogues a chemical memory of the offending pathogen so that it can respond much more quickly when encountering that particular strain of virus again. Without this library of past encounters, we would all be like infants and small children who constantly get sick when exposed to each new virus. But with the **Humoral Immune Response**, we are well-equipped to fend off most colds or flus relatively quickly. The first time your body fights a virus, it can take up to 15 days (or, in some cases, even longer) to generate and complete its complex mission. Because of the **Memory B-cells**, the second time your body sees that virus, the **Humoral Immune Response** can often eliminate the infection in the humors in five days.[23]

While the **B-cell Clone Army** quickly eliminates viruses only in the Humors (or interstitial spaces between the cells), once a virus successfully enters into a cell and infects it, the virus essentially becomes invisible to the **B-cell** system. This is when the **Cell-Mediated Immune Response** becomes critically important, as it helps the body find and fight virus-infected cells. I will review the **Cell-Mediated Immune Response** in detail in the next section.

CELL-MEDIATED IMMUNE RESPONSE

The second part of the **Acquired Immune Response**, the **Cell-Mediated Immune Response**, is entirely controlled and populated by **T-cells**. While the **Cell-Mediated Immune Response** is a unique part of the **Immune Response**, it does have many characteristics that are similar to the capabilities of the **B-cells**. The **T-cells** also have a Janitor function that cleans and eliminates pathogens. Also, like the **B-cells**, there is a sorting process when the matching **T-cell** must be found to bind to a **Macrophage MHC** site. **B-cells** can also display the **MHC** and act as beacons to attract **T-cells** to an infected site.

Like the **B-cells**, these **T-cells** each have a unique binding capability which can be compared to carrying a billion keys on their key ring in order to unlock and bind to the pathogen. After binding to the pathogen, the **T-cells** also raise a **Clone Army** (although in a slightly different way than **B-cells**). Finally, **T-cells** have a **Librarian Army** that functions just like the **B-cell Librarian Army**, only it serves as a memory for the **T-cell**. In fact, both **T-cell** and **B-cell** Librarian Armies are called Memory cells, and these memory cells shorten the process of finding a matching **T-cell** and **B-cells** to bind to the targeted virus and its clones. However, there are important differences between these two systems that we must understand in order to fully comprehend the versatility and synergy of these two systems. We will review the similarities and differences in more depth below.

The first thing that differentiates **T-cells** from **B-cells** is that there are four types of **T-cells** and only two types of **B-cells**. Let's look at these four types of **T-cells**:

1. **T-helper cells**, which activate the production of **B-cell** clones and **T-cell** clones, and also trigger the **B-cells** to produce billions of antibodies. **T-helper cells** also attract **Cytotoxic T-cells** to the infection site.
2. **Cytotoxic T-cells**, which go into an infected cell and kill the virus (as well as the cell) it has hijacked. I call this the **Assassin Army**.
3. **T-Memory cells** form chemical memories of all the viruses that it has encountered and defeated, and can serve as a library to help **B-** and **T-cells** locate the right **B-** and **T-cell** antigens to effectively fight off an identical virus in the future.
4. **T-Regulatory cells**, which turns the volume down once the **Immune Cells** have overcome an attack.

These different types of cells, while important to know, are not helpful in understanding how the **Cell-Mediated Immune Response** works. So let us look functionally at what the **T-cells** can do. After reviewing the functional characteristics of **T-cells**, we can then return to the types of **T-cells** and understand them more completely. We start our exploration with the ability of **T-cells** to eliminate infected cells.

T-cells Can Eliminate Infected Cells

The **T-cells** have some very unique characteristics that differentiate them from **B-cells,** but one of the most important differences lies in the way that they can eliminate viruses from the body. We have learned that **B-cells** can, through their **Clone Army** of antibodies, quickly eliminate pathogens from our system. But this can only happen when those pathogens occupy the intracellular space (the Humors). The problem with viruses is that they actually enter into a cell and in doing so, exit the intracellular fluid. When this happens, the virus becomes invisible to **B-cells**, and **B-cell** antibodies become totally ineffective in eliminating virus-infected cells. As a virus-infected cell also becomes a virus replica factory,[24] the body can soon become overrun by the virus **Clone Army**. Clinical experience has led me to the conclusion that the concentration of this viral storm in the **Second Brain** area, as we discussed in *Chapter 2, Second Brain*, can lead to symptoms of fever, sore throat, as well as suppressed appetite and a depressed mood.

This means that the body must fight off a viral infection on two fronts: one within the humors (intracellular fluid), and one within our cells. While the body ramps up its production of **B-cell** clones and antibodies to fight off the humoral infection, part of the virus escapes into the cells and the **Cellular Immune Response** must also be activated. We will explore just how this **Cellular Immune Response** functions in the next two sections.

T-cell Identification of a Virus

Like **B-cells**, **T-cells** respond to the chemical signal sent by **Macrophages** (and to other cells, including some **B-cells**) and will find and consume virus-infected cells that display **MHC**s on their surface. **T-cells** can only become activated after the **B-cell** cloning. Like **B-cells**, each **T-cell** has a unique receptor and a matching **T-cell** must bind to the **MHC** of the **B-cell** or **Macrophage** that has engulfed a virally-infected cell in order for this **Cellular Immune Response** to actively begin eliminating the infected cells using its cloning capabilities. When the **T-cell** successfully finds and binds to the virally-infected cell, it then begins its own cloning process. The process is a bit slower than **B-cell** cloning, but the result leads to the elimination of the infected cells along with the viral clones that they created.

Programmed Cell Death (The Assassin Army)

The cells that **T-cell** clone once the matching **T-cell** is activated are called **Cytotoxic T-cells**. Using our army analogy, I call these cells the **Assassin Army**. This **Assassin Army** is created much like the **B-cell Clone Army** through a matching **T-cell** with a receptor that binds to an **MHC** from a **Macrophage** or a **B-cell** that has engulfed an infected cell. Once this happens, cloning can be initiated with the help of **T-helper cells** and the process of creating a **Cytotoxic T-cell Clone Army** is created. Like **B-cell** clone armies, **Cytotoxic T-cells** latch on to an **MHC** from a **Macrophage** or a **B-cell** that has engulfed an infected cell relatively quickly and release chemicals that cause program cell death, killing both the virus and the cell it occupies.

Cytotoxic T-cells are like an **Assassin Army** that search and destroy infected cells. As we will learn in *Chapter 1, Highjacked*, viruses completely take over a cell and its component parts so that the entire cell is unrepairable. Once a virus has entered a cell and hijacked the cell's reproductive system, the only way to kill the virus is to also kill the cell it occupies. This is why the process of healing a cold or flu must involve killing off a substantial number of our own infected cells.

The mission of the **Assassin Army** seemingly goes against one of the overarching inner mandates of our **Immune System**: to protect our body, including our cells, from invasion or harm. Using more scientific terminology, the **Immune System** is supposed to differentiate between self and not self. This means that it identifies particles, bacteria and viruses, or other invaders that aren't part of our normal cells or fluid. However, the **Assassin Army** can "see" when one or many of our cells are infected. In a way, an infected cell is a mixture of Self (our own cells) and Not Self (viruses that have taken over our cells). This means that the **Cytotoxic T-cells** can differentiate between a healthy cell and a diseased cell, and can help eliminate a viral infection even though the infection is in our own cells. There is a kind of intelligence to the **Assassin Army** in that they are able to differentiate problems that are hidden from virtually all of the rest of the **Immune Response**.

Once the **Cytotoxic T-cells** have eliminated all the infected cells, then the body must stop creating the **Cytotoxic T-cells** and, over time, shift into creating new cells to replace the ones that have been killed off and clean up the debris left in the wake of the clone war.[25] The cloning of virally-infected cells along with **B-cells** and **Cytotoxic T-cells** leading to infection and the killing of millions of viruses and virally-infected cells along with the recreating of new healthy cells may be one of the reasons that most people become tired and listless in virtually all stages of colds or flus. However, being tired and listless and enduring uncomfortable symptoms is a small price to pay as these **Acquired Immune Cells** serve as one of the keys to our survival and stand as a monument to the resourcefulness of our **Immune Response**.

T-Memory Cells

T-Memory cells form a chemical memory of each particular virus that infected us. It is these cells, along with **B-Memory cells**, that provide the key differentiating factor between the **Acquired Immune System** and the **Innate Immune System**. **Memory Cells** are able to "acquire" a living memory of a conquered viral infection as well as maintain a "library" of all infections we've encountered. I call these cells the **Librarian Army** and this division of cells is created at the same time that the **Cytotoxic T-cells** clones are formed. That means that they hold a memory of the **Cytotoxic T-cells** that cloned and defeated the cold or flu virus. Because of this **Librarian Army**, our **T-Memory Cells** can assist the **Cytotoxic T-cells** more quickly find and bind to any cold viruses we've been infected with in the past. This provides an important short cut for our **Immune Response**, and means that the matching **Cytotoxic T-cells** can more quickly be created to quell the infection.

Librarian Army cells, once created, remain in our system for years and often decades after an infection is quelled and become part of a living library that the **T-cells** system can access whenever we encounter an identical virus infection. This applies to the **B-cell Librarian Army** as well. Because of **T-Memory cells**, our **Immune Response** can utilize this function far more efficiently and help the body conserve resources whenever we get infected by a virus we've encountered in the past.

Infants start out their life with an empty library. However, with each cold or flu they catch, their library begins to fill with a larger and larger array of **T-Memory cells** that can match up a correct **Cytotoxic T-cell** to similar future viral infections. On a practical level, it means that infants and small children have no, or at least very few, **B-** or **T-Memory cells** circulating in their bloodstream.

T-cells as the Regulators of the Immune Response

The final type of **T-cells** are called **T-Regulatory**. These, along with the **T-helper cells**, are a kind of command center that both help to rally the **Acquired Immune Response** when we catch a cold or flu and lower the **Immune Response** once the virus causing the cold or flu is conquered. **T-helper cells** help to initiate the **T-cell** and **B-cell** cloning while **T-Regulatory** help to restore our **Immune System** to its basic surveillance function. The **T-helper cells** and **T-Regulatory** are the regulators of the **Immune Response**.

While the **T-Regulatory Cells** are critical to turning the **Immune Response** down, often their actions lag behind the quelling of the infection. This means that the symptoms associated with the ending of a cold of flu usually persist for a few days even though the **T-cells** have successfully eliminated the virus and all its clones. Of course, this means that the process of healing from a cold or flu can take more time; sometimes up to a week or more as the **Immune Response** slowly normailizes. As we will learn in *Chapter 5, EliminatingYour Cough by Clearing Out Clutter* and *Chapter 7, Let the Acetylcholine Flow*, herbal medicine and other natural therapies can assist in speeding up this winding down of the cold symptoms while lessening the effects of the end of cold symptoms.[26]

We can now see the Innate and **Acquired Immune Response** working together to help protect our body from viruses and other pathogens. Without **Macrophages** and other cells within the **Innate Immune Response**, **MHC**'s would not be created and the infection would be invisible to the **Acquired Immune Response**. Likewise, without the **Acquired Immune Response**, the identification, cloning of **T-Cytotoxic** and storing of information to help with future infections through **T-Memory cells** would not be possible. But all of these astounding defenses would be pointless without the command function of the **T-Regulatory** and **T-helper cells** which serve to regulate the overall **Immune Response**. Afterall, without the **T-Regulatory**, we might find ourselves having a perpetual fever. which would be extremely depleting our inner resources and energy.

The Shortcomings of the T-cell System

The **T-cell** collection of fighters, regulators and librarians is the most sophisticated part of our **Immune System**, effectively protecting us from all but the most virulent invaders. However, the **T-cells** cellular immune system has an inherent weakness of which we should be aware. This weakness has to do with the time it takes for the matching **T-cell** to find the **MHC** that is being displayed by the **Macrophages** or **B-cells**. In fact, it often takes a week or two for the **T-cells** to gear up, find the right match and produce the millions of clones needed to fight a virally-infected cell.

To review the process:

1. Locate the infection with the help of the **MHCs** in **Macrophages** and **B-cells**.
2. Once the matching **T-cell** is found, **T-helper cells** along with **Cytokines** must initiate the cloning process.
3. Then they must engage the **T-suppressor-cells** to tamp down the **Immune Response**.

Nevertheless, without **T-cells**, our system is ill-equipped to effectively kill virus-infected cells. Along with their ability to modulate the **Immune Response**, **T-cells** provide a critically important component of the **Immune System** that contributes immeasurably to our well-being and longevity.

All this shows that all parts of our **Immune System** work in concert to provide comprehensive protection from most viruses. It also highlights the real importance of maintaining a strong **T-cell** system as the **T-helper Cells** are responsible for turning on and activating **B-cells** to produce antibodies, as well as activating **Cytotoxic T-cells**. I am reviewing the **Immune Response** in order to explain an herbal approach to activate the **Immune Response**, but we must first look at one more immune cell that is critical to the immune function: the **Natural Killer Cell**.

NATURAL KILLER CELLS – OUR IMMUNE SYSTEM'S ULTIMATE SECRET WEAPON

Now that we have an overview of our **Immune System** and how the **Innate** and **Cell-Mediated Immune Response** works, we can look at the final piece of the puzzle: the **Natural Killer Cell** (**NK cell**). **NK cells** are another **Assassin Cell Army**, often providing a vital shortcut to the complex process of mounting an effective defense against a cold or flu virus. However, unlike **Cytotoxic T-cells** or **B-cells, NK cells** do not require the tedious process of sorting and matching up of the **MHCs** on **Macrophages** and **B-cells**. Instead, they have the ability to find and kill off virally-infected cells whenever they encounter them. We could say that both **B-cells** and **Cytotoxic T-cells** are blind armies that need **MHCs** in order to find the infection, while **NK cells** are capable of finding and killing infected-cells all on their own without any of the complex sorting and matching.

While **NK cells** have long been recognized as capable of killing virally-infected cells just like **Cytotoxic T-cells**, **NK cells** have, until recently, been assigned to the **Innate Immune System** as they "rapidly respond against target cells in the absence of prior sensitization (meaning they have no **NK Memory Cells**), as well as because of the previous belief that they are cells with a short lifespan."[27] Information in the past few years has yielded a new understanding of these extraordinary cells because, like a **Cell-Mediated Immune Response**, they provide potent chemicals that can easily destroy a virally-infected cell. In other words, they share characteristics of the **Innate** and the **Cell-Mediated Immune Response**.

For this reason, **NK cells** have experienced a resurgence of research. In fact, "**NK cells** are of considerable interest for immunotherapy, since they manifest cytotoxic activity against virus-infected and tumor cells."[28] Moreover, they do not require the complex and time-consuming identification and cloning that **B-cells** or **T-cells** require to find and attack the virus infection. As we will see, this immune cell can be stimulated using herbal medicine and speed the course of your recovery while lessening the severity of your symptoms.

NK Cell Limitations

We must understand that, while **NK cells** share the same lethal power to eliminate virally- infected cells as **Cytotoxic T-cells**, they have some limitations that must be addressed to make them an effective weapon when activated to fight a viral cold or flu. The main limitation is that they cannot create a **Clone Army** like **B-** and **T-cells** and, therefore, are unable to create sufficient numbers to mount an effective viral attack. This whole process is like a cloning war with millions of soldiers on each side. However, with the aid of herbal medicine, particularly medicinal mushrooms and other natural supplements, this limitation can be overcome.

This is very good news for those who want to skip over the time-consuming process that is required by the **Cell-Mediated Immune Response** led by **B-** and **T-cells**. Instead, medical mushrooms can accomplish the same job. However, this ramping up of **NK cell** populations appears to temporarily stimulate increased numbers through cytokine (chemical) stimulation, but only for 1 to 3 hours.[29] For this reason dosing every 1 to 2 hours is necessary to maintain a high level of **NK cells** so that they have sufficient numbers to quell the virus replication and expansion. If the populations of these unique cytotoxic cells plummet, the virus can then reassert its viral cloning machines and overwhelm the healing that the medicinal herbs had begun.

In this stage of the virus, I usually recommend frequent dosing of herbal therapies to support the **Immune Response**. For more specific treatment options and dosing recommendations, please refer to the last section of this chapter. If you wish to read more about this herbal approach, there is a lot of research that documents the effective **Cell-Mediated** response of medicinal mushrooms. Please note that most of the research about mushrooms documents its positive effect on another health issue that benefits from **Cell-Mediated** response, cancer. Because mushrooms may have healing properties for cancer, there has been a lot of research conducted over the past 20 years.[30] By happy accident, this aids in my quest to find the ultimate weapon to fight cold and flu viruses.

PROBLEMS THAT OVERSTRESS OR INTERFERE WITH THE IMMUNE SYSTEM

Before we review therapeutic interventions such as acupuncture, herbs and supplements, let's talk about the problems that prevent the **Immune System** from functioning optimally. These problems, listed below, either suppress or overwork the **Immune Response**. This section will address medications, health conditions, vulnerable populations, and finally, environmental concerns. It is quite important to review these problems as these factors can interfere with the healing process even if you diligently follow an herbal protocol.

Below are the factors that can interfere with our healing.

MEDICATIONS

There are many medications that interfere with immune function. In this section, I will list some of the most common ones and how, if possible, to mitigate these problems.

Prednisone and Cortisone

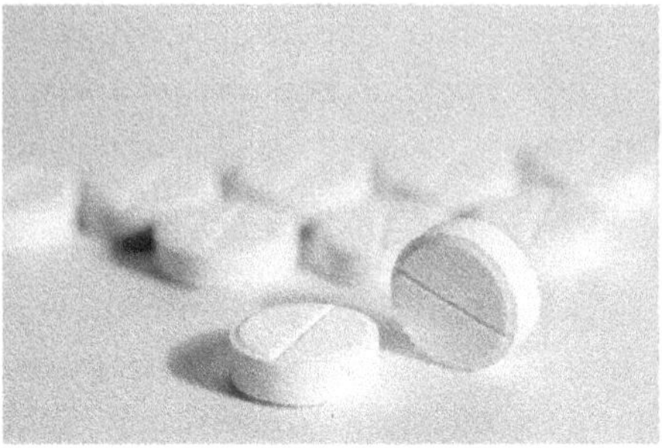

Prednisone and Cortisone are medicines that were first developed in the 1950s and have widely been considered the most powerful anti-inflammatory drugs available to this day. These medicines can offer a valuable tool for modern medicine to help patients with extreme pain who need to manage a chronic health condition. However, these drugs come with very significant side effects that should be weighed carefully before anyone considers taking them. These side effects are so severe that at one point both of these medicines were temporarily taken off the market in order for drug companies to recalibrate appropriate dosages and restrictions. Although now widely available, it is common knowledge that these side effects include kidney damage and osteoporosis along with a whole host of other problematic negative effects. Perhaps one of the most ironic and confusing therapeutic actions that Prednisone or **Cortisol** exerts on the body is that it actually suppresses the **Immune Response.**[31]

It may be obvious why suppressing the **Immune Response** may be a bad idea, especially to those who have read this chapter on the **Immune System**. However, in certain circumstances, suppressing the **Immune Response** may provide a life-saving miracle for someone who has extreme pain. Most pain is the result of an inflammatory condition such as severe arthritis, bursitis, or traumatic injury. However, by suppressing the **Immune Response**, these medications also leave the patient more vulnerable to catching an infection, including a cold or flu virus.

The myriad of ways that Prednisone and **Cortisol** suppress the **Immune Response** is complex, but it is clear that these drugs suppress many parts of the **Immune Response**, including parts of the **Innate Immune Response** like the **Dendritic Immune Cells**. This can complicate a patient's ability to fight off infections like an **ENS cold** or flu. Prednisone and **Cortisol** also suppress other parts of the Innate and **Acquired Immune Response** as they suppress the overall production of **White blood cells** including **Macrophages, B-cells** and **T-cells.**[32]

New evidence also suggests that Prednisone and **Cortisol** have a significant adverse effect on the **Gut Microbiome.**[33] This alone would raise concern for those who wish to preserve their digestive function as these effects may last long after a patient has stopped taking this medicine. In addition to this deleterious effect on the **Gut Microbiome**, drugs in this family of anti-inflammatories have also been shown to adversely affect gut permeability.[34] The common name for this problem is "**Leaky Gut Syndrome**" and this gut issue leads to an elevated **Immune Response** which, like so many other issues we are discussing, taxes the **Immune System** and ultimately can lead to a less vital **Immune Response** for fighting off a cold or flu.

Today, viable and effective alternatives to these drugs often provide a healthier means to finding pain relief while providing a more viable, long-term pathway to healing. Acupuncture now stands as a leading alternative approach backed up by major studies.[35,36] In fact the American College of Physicians now recommends Acupuncture along with superficial heat, massage and spinal manipulation as first-line protocols for the treatment of low back pain.[37,38]

If using alternative approaches are not possible and you cannot reduce or stop utilizing these medicines, then my recommendation is to take probiotics to help mitigate **Gut Microbiome** and **Leaky Gut** issues and, to the degree that your are able, maintain at least a minimal exercise routine. Managing stress is also very important for those who are on Prednisone for more than a few weeks as Cortisone is a precursor to **Cortisol**, which is one of the two principal stress hormones. Elevated **Cortisol**, as we will learn in *Chapter 4, The Body's Secret Regulator*, indicates that one's system is under greater effects of stress. Exercise helps to restore balance to this hormone and can thereby reduce its deleterious effects. Refer to *Chapter 4, The Body's Secret Regulator* for more specific details on how to effectively manage stress.

Antibiotics

Antibiotics have a direct and sometimes significantly negative effect on the **Gut Microbiome**. Many patients find that taking antibiotics results in stomach pain, diarrhea and/or constipation and sometimes can lead to a chronic condition such as **Irritable Bowel Syndrome** (IBS), Crohns, or Fibromyalgia. Besides the **Gut Microbiome**, antibiotics also can suppress **Lymphocyte** (another term for **White blood cells**) transformation and can suppress antibody production.[39] For most people, finding an alternative to antibiotics or at least taking probiotics daily is important.

NSAIDS

Any anti-inflammatory medication like Ibuprofen and Motrin will, over time, interfere with the stomach and intestine's ability to manufacture the mucosal lining. This can lead, within weeks or months depending on the person, to stomach and intestinal problems such as Chronic Gastritis, **Silent Reflux**, or Intestinal Dysbiosis. These are not isolated or rare problems and we now find that these problems are documented by current research.[40] These problems can lead to chronic inflammation and thus, over time, result in overtaxing the **Immune Response**.

In addition to the thinning of the mucosal lining, NSAIDS can ultimately cause **GERD** or **Silent Reflux**, which almost always results in the irritation of the stomach lining causing inflammation at the junction of the **Lower Esophageal Valve**. Therefore, patients with **GERD** or **Silent Reflux** usually have a greater chance of catching a cold and, once they catch a cold or flu, have a harder time recovering. For someone who has **GERD** or **Silent Reflux**, I usually recommend Slippery Elm, which can be found as a main ingredient in many cough drops, teas or herbal supplements. This safe, herbal medicine should be continued for at least a few weeks or until all of the **GERD** or **Silent Reflux** symptoms abate.

Chemotherapy

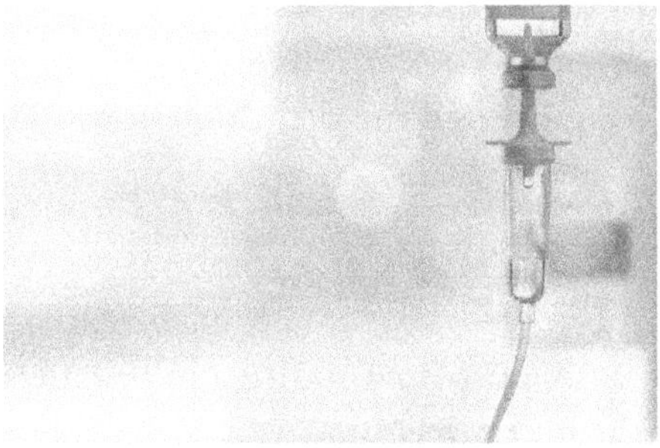

Chemotherapy drugs often suppress the **Immune Response**. In fact, chemotherapy must sometimes be temporarily stopped if the **White Blood Cell** (**WBC**) count becomes too low. **WBC** is a broad generic term that means **Immune Cells**.
Taking probiotics and stomach-soothing herbs such as Slippery Elm can help mitigate some of the harsh effects of chemotherapy and help to restore immune function. Research also indicates that Astragalus, a Chinese herb, can be helpful in restoring **WBC** levels more quickly.[41]

Humira® and Other Autoimmune Medications that Suppress the Immune Response

Autoimmune Medicines like Humira® work by suppressing parts of the **Immune Response**. This, in turn, provides symptom relief from chronic pain associated with autoimmune diseases such as Rheumatoid Arthritis. I often suggest that patients try acupuncture and herbal and/or diet therapy as a way to reduce or eliminate pain as well as their prescribed immune-suppressing medicines. Acupuncture and herbs do require ongoing treatment, but do not suppress the **Immune Response**. These health issues can be complex and often require a pain management program directed by a skilled alternative healthcare professional.

HEALTH CONDITIONS THAT OVERTAX THE IMMUNE SYSTEM

These conditions may include:

- Chronic back pain.
- Chronic neck pain or whiplash.
- Osteoarthritis.
- Rheumatoid arthritis.
- Chronic tendonitis.
- Rotator cuff strains.
- Chronic bursitis.
- Fibromyalgia.
- Plantar fasciitis.
- Chronic headaches or migraines.
- Lupus.
- Sciatica.
- Neuropathy.
- Any other chronic pain condition.

Any of these conditions can generate a considerable amount of inflammation, which can trigger a substantial **Immune Response**. The **Immune Response** responds to injury similar to how it treats a pathogen, working to reduce inflammation and promote tissue healing. If untreated, a painful condition can result in the **Immune System**'s response becoming more muted and less effective. The **Acquired Immune Response** becomes particularly depleted so that as a patient's pain condition progresses, the body's ability to appropriately respond declines.

Natural approaches to these problems, such as Acupuncture, Herbal Therapy and Osteopathic Manual Medicine, work alongside Physical Therapy and Massage and can offer a slow but effective way to gradually reduce inflammation and thereby help to restore the immune function.

Stress

For an in-depth understanding of how stress affects the **Immune Response**, please refer to the chapter on stress as this is a complex and multifaceted problem that creates a myriad of problems for the **Immune Response**.

Problems Caused by an Unhealthy Gut Microbiome

Anyone who suffers with **Irritable Bowel Syndrome** (IBS), Crohn's Disease, chronic gas and bloating, or chronic constipation is also overtaxing the **Immune Response**. Research informs us that these problems are frequently the result of the **Gut Microbiome** being out of balance.[42] **Gut Microbiome** problems are typically due to an overgrowth of unhealthy bacteria, fungus, or parasites, all of which cause chronic swelling, inflammation and irregular bowel movements along with additional effects of **Leaky Gut Syndrome**.

Gut Microbiome can, over time, overburden the **Immune Response** and lead to a worsening of these conditions. Probiotics and restricting one's diet from **Gut Microbiome** problem foods such as sugar and starches can help to reduce unhealthy populations within the gut and can help to restore balance to the **Gut Microbiome**.

Gut Microbiome problems also interfere directly with the **Immune System**. In fact, new research demonstrates that an unhealthy **Gut Microbiota** can lead to inhibiting the **Immune System**'s ability to produce **T-Regulatory** and **T-helper cells**. This points to broad-reaching effects that can have a profound effect on our health in many ways. Equally troubling are new discoveries that reveal that a healthy **Gut Microbiome** stimulates **Cytokines** that trigger the release of **T-Regulatory Cells** and **Th17 Cells**.[43] (**Th17 Cells** are one of the activating chemicals that stimulate **NK cells**.) This means an unhealthy **Gut Microbiome** may inhibit the release of these vital **Cytokines** and thereby disable an important part of our **Immune Response**.

Another way an unhealthy **Gut Microbiome** is leading to serious health concerns is with an elevation of pro-inflammatory cells.[44] The implications of this discovery means that those who have an unhealthy **Gut Microbiome** will have more problems regulating their **Immune Response**. Many find themselves chronically inflamed with a disabled **Immune Response** resulting in compromised immunity and again, more vulnerable to catching colds with a weaker **Immune System** to fight them.

Like many chronic conditions, these problems often require the guidance of a skilled alternative healthcare practitioner who can provide the testing and nutritional guidance that is needed.

Chronic Gastritis, GERD and Silent Reflux

If your stomach is inflamed due to an ulcer or you have acid reflux (**GERD**), an inflammatory burden is put on the **Immune System** which will, over time, weaken the **Immune Response**. (**Silent Reflux** is a milder version of **GERD** with more subtle symptoms.) Also, because many colds originate from this area which is, in fact, traversed by the **Enteric Nervous System**, an inflamed stomach or **GERD** situation can present a double or triple burden to the **Immune Response**. As we will learn in *Chapter 4, The Body's Secret Regulator*, inflammation can activate the **Sympathetic Stress Response**, shunting blood flow away from the GI organs to the extremities. The **Sympathetic Stress Response** can amplify the inflammatory burden and overtax the **Immune Response** even more quickly. Sometimes this complex problem can be alleviated by simply taking Slippery Elm, which can help with stomach issues such as these. Of course, if this doesn't resolve your heart burn, you may need to seek the guidance of a holistic health practitioner.

Osteoporosis

Recently, research has revealed that there is a strong correlation between the health of the bones and bone-remodeling systems and our immunity. This connection is so important that a new development of an interdisciplinary branch of medicine called Osteoimmunology has been established in order to study this fascinating connection.[45] In a recent paper, scientists summarized the correlation between Osteoclasts (which break down old bone) and Osteoblasts (which build new bone). "...[O]steoclasts, the bone-resorbing cells, are derived from the same myeloid precursor cells that give rise to **Macrophages** and myeloid dendritic cells. On the other hand, osteoblasts, the bone-forming cells, regulate hematopoietic stem cell niches from which all blood and **Immune Cells** are derived."[46]

Osteoporosis is an extremely common condition. Most menopausal women suffer from a progressive thinning of the bones which is the main symptom of Osteoporosis. Complementary and Alternative Medicine (**CAM**) has helped many patients to formulate natural supplements to help with this problem. As an aside, men are not immune to Osteoporosis and so they, too, should be evaluated by their physicians for this condition.

Toxins

The toxic burden of our modern world is increasing as industrial waste keeps finding its way into our streams and oceans which then affects our water and food. There are two main categories of toxins that have a direct impact on our immune function. The first is an increased load of **Organophosphates** and **Organochlorines**, which include many pesticides, herbicides, and PCPs as well as tailpipe pollution. Each of these are chemically similar enough to **Estrogen** that these chemicals can bind to our body's **Estrogen** sites. The result as we grow older is that these chemicals can accumulate and elevate **Estrogen** levels.

Even natural **Estrogen** is undesirable when the body produces too much. But these chemical **Estrogen**-like substances are more challenging for the body to get rid of and can lead to unhealthy levels of more dangerous subtypes of **Estrogen**. The medical term for this elevation of **Estrogen** (no matter which type) is called **Estrogen Dominance**. This is problematic for many reasons. For one, it can lead to premature menopause or more pronounced PMS symptoms. Moreover, **Organophosphates** and **Organochlorines** can lead to additional problems such as the increased risk of breast and uterine cancer.[47]

At the very least, **Estrogen Dominance** can increase inflammation in the body,[48] which again increases the burden on the **Immune System**, leaving us more vulnerable to colds and flus. For those who wish to lessen the **Organophosphate** and **Organochlorine** burden, moving to less polluted areas or, at minimum, increasing cruciferous vegetables can help the body break down these chemicals.[49] Equally important is eating a higher percentage of organic vegetables and fruits, and drinking filtered water. These two measures can greatly help to minimize this health risk.

The second toxic burden is heavy metals. In my view, heavy metals are one of the most hidden, yet important public health issues of our time. Many heavy metals, like Mercury, Cadmium and Arsenic, are actual poisons that suppress and/or kill cells in our bodies, including **Immune Cells**. It should not be surprising that heavy metals are infiltrating our food chain as mercury is now widely acknowledged as a problem that is present in much of the fish that we eat.[50] The fish shown to have the highest levels of Mercury include:

- Mackerel (King).
- Marlin.
- Orange Roughy.
- Shark.
- Swordfish.
- Tilefish.
- Tuna (Bigeye, Ahi).[51]

Not only is Mercury on everyone's radar these days, Arsenic is also entering the spotlight. It seems that there are high levels of residual Arsenic embedded in much of the soil where rice is grown in America, especially in the southern states where so much of America's rice is grown. Arsenic, like Mercury, should be monitored, especially if you eat rice. Cadmium and Lead are also common enough to warrant getting a comprehensive test that includes all four. Research suggests that heavy metals, even in small doses, can induce or inhibit **B-cells** as well as many **Innate Immune Cells** and **Cytokines**.

While not everyone has heavy metal toxicity, if you have chronic health problems that are not responding to alternative or conventional treatment, you should probably have your heavy metal load tested. Please note that not all detoxification methods are effective. Even if you are taking precautions against heavy metal toxicity, you may still suffer from exposure and a build up of one or more heavy metals in your system. In recent years, I have become more aware of how damaging even mild heavy metal toxicity can be, no matter how many great supplements we take or how much exercise we get.

People that have a toxic burden of heavy metals need help to find safe ways to remove them. I prefer methods that are currently being developed by Dr. Christopher W. Shade.[52] Dr. Shade is considered a leading expert in heavy metal detection and treatment, and has developed more advanced testing and elimination protocols.

I recommend that patients get tested if they report any of the following symptoms:

1. **GERD** or **Silent Reflux** symptoms without any physical cause such as a hiatal hernia or ulcers that do not fully respond to proton-pump inhibitors, acupuncture treatment, or botanicals such as Slippery Elm.
2. Hard and/or swollen abdomen.
3. Episodic stomach cramps.
4. Chronic fatigue symptoms without an anemia or hypothyroidism diagnosis.
5. A growing list of foods that trigger allergy-like symptoms.
6. Poor sleep or insomnia, especially with restlessness.
7. Chronic skin rashes.
8. Sudden development of an autoimmune disease like Hashimoto's Thyroiditis, Rheumatoid Arthritis, Lupus, Sjogren's or Fibromyalgia.
9. Unexplained increased liver enzymes, Kidney Creatinine or GFR levels.

To be very clear, just because someone has one or more of these symptoms does not necessarily mean that they suffer from heavy metal toxicity. Toxicity is only one possible diagnosis that should be ruled in or out.

Toxicity is a growing concern as our soil and oceans are becoming more and more polluted. As our pollution load increases, it's clear that our **Immune Systems** are having to work overtime, leaving us more vulnerable to catching a cold.

Summary: An Overtaxed Immune Function

If your **Immune System** is overtaxed, the main consequence is that you will be more likely to catch frequent colds or flus, as well as other infections. If you catch colds frequently, then you should review this chapter carefully and take note of any health conditions that you have or medications that you're taking that increase your vulnerability. You may need to consult with a qualified healthcare professional. The last section of this chapter will be important for you to review as you will find that there are several potent, natural solutions to help boost your **Immune Response**.

The truth is, even if you have a robust **Immune System**, or just a normal **Immune System** where you catch just one or two colds a year, you should still consider using the immune boosting strategies that I list as it will, at a minimum, significantly lessen the duration of a cold or flu.

NATURAL METHODS TO BOOST YOUR IMMUNE SYSTEM

There are three powerful natural methods for boosting your **Immune Response**:

1. Medicinal Mushrooms.
2. Probiotics.
3. Acupuncture.

Medicinal Mushrooms

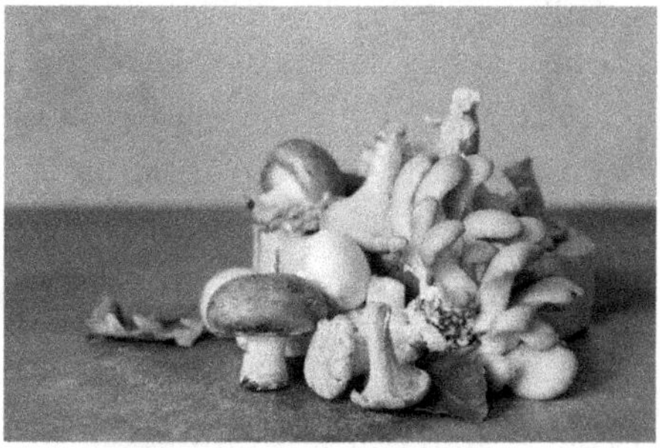

According to the latest medical research, the most powerful way to stimulate the **Immune Response** using natural methods is by using medicinal mushrooms. Mushrooms provide a powerful immune-modulating effect which helps to tamp down the **Innate Immune Response** while stimulating the cellular defense system within the **Acquired Immune Response**.

Let us quickly look at what science has revealed about how medicinal mushrooms mount an effective **Immune Response** to catching a cold.

Tamping Down the Innate Immune System

The **Innate Immune System** stimulates a pro-inflammatory generic response to an infection, creating inflammation and fever (along with swelling and pain) to begin the fight to help the body fend off a viral infection. The **Innate Immune Response**, however, contributes little towards winning the battle against a viral cold except that it, after many days, can act as a beacon that alerts the **Acquired Immune Response** and helps present the virus in a form that **T-cells** and **NK cells** can recognize. While your system is sorting through millions of cells, this Innate Response is creating most of your symptoms, including a sore throat, fever, a stuffy or runny nose, and lethargy. Tamping down this Innate Response can help reduce the severity of your symptoms.

Scientists measure how active the Innate System is by evaluating how the **Immune System** is modulated by a therapeutic agent. If, for instance, the overall effect reduces inflammation, calming the **Innate Immune Response**, it is called a TH1. On the other hand, TH2 indicates the opposite, that the **Immune System** is more proinflammatory. Research now shows that medicinal mushrooms increase TH1 and decrease TH2. This increase in TH1 and decrease in TH2 shown when using medicinal mushrooms means that medicinal mushrooms are anti-inflammatory agents.

Cordyceps is an example of a mushroom that helps reduce the pro-inflammatory effects of the **Innate Immune Response**. In a recent study, scientists found that an extract of Cordyceps increases TH1 activity and decreases TNF-a (a pro-inflammatory Innate Immune Cell), as well as other pro-inflammatory **Cytokines.**[53] Other mushrooms that also increased TH1, include Agaricus[54,55], Reishi[56,57,58,59,60], Maitake[61,62,63,64,65,66,67,68], and Turkey Tail.[69,70,71]

Even though this is an impressive finding, if this was the only effect that medicinal mushrooms had, they would be of little value in treating a cold. They would only serve to suppress the **Immune System**, albeit, the most pro-inflammatory part of it. If this were the case, medicinals mushrooms would provide temporary relief followed by an exacerbation of the viral infection. In the next section we will examine the effect they also have on the **Acquired Immune Response**.

Activating the Acquired Immune Response

The most beneficial effect of medicinal mushrooms is in their ability to activate the **Acquired Immune Response**. Science has much to learn about the intricacies of how these mushrooms amplify the **Acquired Immune Response**, but we already know that they stimulate the production of both **Cytotoxic T-cells** and **NK cells**. This fact is one of the reasons why scientists are studying medicinal mushrooms so diligently. These cells not only help effectively fight off a cold or flu, but also help the body mount an attack against certain cancers. While the verdict regarding how much they help with the fight against cancer is, at this time, unclear (but promising), this research now helps us to understand much more about why mushrooms help the body fight off colds or flu so effectively.

The most important **Acquired Immune Cells** that medicinal mushrooms help to stimulate are the **NK cells**, which are the secret weapon of the **Immune System** as they do not need a particular binding site configuration to bind to a virally-infected cell's **MHC** as **Cytotoxic T-cells** do. Recent studies show that many medicinal mushrooms do stimulate the production of **NK cells**. Mushrooms such as Agaricus,[72] Reishi,[73,74,75,76] Maitake,[77] Turkey Tail,[78] and Chaga Mushrooms.[79,80]

We can now see why taking medicinal mushrooms might be an effective means of reducing the intensity and duration of a cold or flu.

Medicinal mushroom include:

- Reishi (Ganoderma).
- Lion's Mane.
- Turkey Tail.
- Shiitake.
- Cordyceps.
- Chaga.

Teas, liquids or pills from reputable companies offer a simple but effective herbal approach to boost immunity. It is generally advised to follow the directions on the label of the product. However, for an active cold or flu, mushrooms must be taken far more frequently and in greater quantity than the label may indicate. For instance, I usually recommend taking the recommended dosage and increase the frequency. For someone experiencing the descent into a cold or flu, I may recommend taking 3 to 4 tablets of an herbal mixture once an hour until the intensity of the symptoms subsides. This may mean that a person will be taking hourly doses for 6 to 8 hours.

When symptoms such as a sore throat and fatigue begin to abate, I recommend reducing the frequency to every 2 to 4 hours. The use of frequent dosing should be considered only during the most acute period of a cold or flu and should not be continued for more than a day or two.

Side Effects

All of the mushrooms listed above have been used medicinally and for culinary purposes for thousands of years, and side effects associated with them are considered rare and are usually mild. Reishi has been catalogued as "Class 1: Herbs that can be safely consumed when used appropriately." This means that it has been scientifically validated as safe. Other mushrooms listed here have more generic warnings which means you should stop taking mushrooms, or any other herb, if it causes generalized itching, indigestion or nausea, or any other negative effect.

Probiotics

Probiotics have been proven to boost the **Immune Response** and help speed the healing process of a common cold or flu. The prestigious *Cochrane Review* in "12 Randomized Controlled Trials" states that "Probiotics were found to be better than placebo in reducing the number of participants experiencing episodes of acute URTI by about 47% and the duration of an episode of acute URTI by about 1.89 days."[81,82] Which probiotics are most effective in supporting immune function? Science is starting to provide answers for us. For instance, Lactobacillus rhamnosus GG.[83,84] In general, I've found a broad spectrum probiotic with at least 25 billion bacteria per pill to be effective. Also I have found refrigerated probiotics tend to be far more potent and effective.

Acupuncture

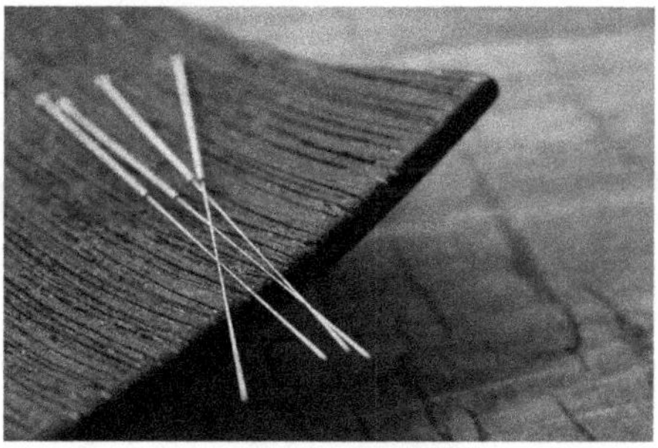

Acupuncture can offer remarkable relief with just a few treatments for conditions such as a stiff neck or any pain condition. For more biomechanical, pain-related problems Cupping Therapy as well as Osteopathic or Chiropractic adjustments can be extremely helpful. Massage can offer some relief as well, although massage alone often is not sufficient for chronic pain conditions. Physical therapy and other exercise specialties can often help to strengthen the body after pain-related treatment are sufficiently healed to ensure that the body becomes hardened and more resistant to re-injury. Additionally, there is now evidence that acupuncture stimulates blood flow as well as **T-cell** and **NK cell** production.[85,86,87] This means that acupuncture can serve as a therapy to reduce inflammation, including the **ENS**, as well as the neck and sinuses. A typical common cold treatment will include needles for at least half an hour in the upper stomach region. Typical acupuncture points should include the following points:

Acupuncture Treatments Protocol for Common Cold

ENS COLD OR FLU	TIGHT NECK	FEVER
Stomach 21, 22	Small Intestine 4	LI 11
Ren 14, 13	Urinary Bladder 64	
Cervical manual traction		

Other acupuncture treatments can be found in chapters relating to specific problems, such as a cough or a sinus infection.

Other Botanical and Nutrients that Might Help the Immune Response

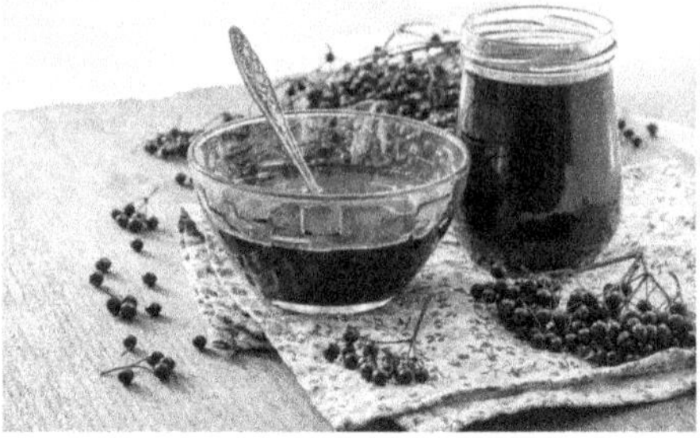

Zinc

There is some evidence that Zinc can assist in helping the body maintain **NK cells** and **T-helper cell** populations.[88]

Elderberry

Elderberry is not an herbal remedy that I have used with my patients, but I do have some patients who report a lessening of cold symptoms and cold duration while using it. It has some promising research that shows that it can be used against flus and colds.[89]

Echinacea

Echinacea is definitely in the top 10 most studied herbs in the world. However, there are nine different species of Echinacea which all have different phytochemicals. According to experts in the herbal field, alkamides found in some species are considered the most likely key ingredient. If this is the case, then this means that extracting Echinacea in water or simply taking it in a tea form are unlikely to reap any benefit. On the other hand, even for properly extracted herbs that are appropriately utilized and dosed, the results are not impressive. In fact, there is some evidence that Echinacea has a weak effect on our Immune Function that may only help some. The *Cochrane Review*'s conclusion is that the results are mixed with only a possible mild effect in enhancing Immune Function. Having said that, I have encountered patients that have received good results from using Echinacea. If you choose to try Echinacea, I would recommend an alcohol tincture or a very mild infusion of fresh Echinacea flowers.

Vitamin D

People with low levels of Vitamin D are more likely to catch a cold. I have not included Vitamin D in my top recommendations as it stands more as a preventative measure and only helps those whose levels are low. It is worth noting, medicinal mushrooms are very high in Vitamin D.

SEEKING PROFESSIONAL HELP

All of these strategies can offer powerful assistance in reducing the intensity and duration of a cold. It is often advisable to work with a professional as you navigate through this rather complex world of herbs and alternative treatments. Choosing the right herbs along with their dosage can be paramount in having a successful outcome. Acupuncture, which is an optional treatment, can be helpful, but in my estimation, herbal treatments are critically important.

After many years of refining my treatments through the review of current research and from the insights gained from treating hundreds of patients with colds and flus, I have learned that frequent dosing of herbs is often crucial. Moreover, finding someone who is comfortable stepping away from traditional Traadional Chinese Medicine-styled diagnosis to treat using Western research can save patients a lot of frustration. There are certain exceptions to the rules. For instance, if you have a summer heat cold (alternating fever and chills, some diarrhea, a frontal headache and a stuffy head), I believe that you will be better off with a traditional Chinese herbal mixture like Huo Xiang Zheng Qi Teng rather than following the protocol shown above.

The following chapters will deal with specific problems associated with the common cold and flu. Stress, coughs, and sinus infections are addressed in the upcoming chapters.

CHAPTER 4

The Body's Secret Regulator: How to Restore Vagal Tone and Combat Stress Related to Your Cold or Flu

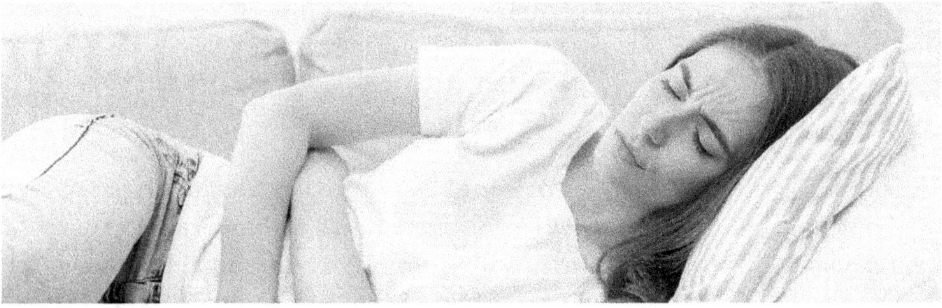

Stress creates many significant health challenges. However, the focus of this chapter is to examine how, when we're stressed, we are more likely to catch a cold or flu. Much has been discovered about the nature of stress and how to combat it in the past few years, shedding light on how stress works and how it affects so much of our mental and physical health. In this chapter, we will explore the many causes of stress and provide appropriate solutions that can help you deal with it more effectively and, in the process, lessen the impact it has on your immunity, helping your body more effectively combat colds and flus. In the first section of this chapter, I will look at what is called top-down **Stress Response**. Top-down stress refers to stress generated by our perceptions and psychological reactions to life's challenges. In the second section, I will review more recent discoveries that outline a bottom-up **Stress Response** which looks at chronic inflammation as a stressor.

WHAT IS STRESS?

To the casual observer, the symptoms of a stressed person, experiencing any number of life challenges, can appear almost invisible. Nevertheless, there are many physical and psychological signs and symptoms of stress which are more than apparent to a qualified healthcare provider. The most common can include fatigue, tense muscles (especially the shoulders and neck), and, in more extreme stress, insomnia, stomach pain, nausea, chest pain, and/or a rapid heartbeat. Even feeling mildly depressed or anxious can be a symptom associated with stress. A person suffering from significant stress can almost always feel one or more of these symptoms. Of course, the tendency to catch colds more frequently is also a symptom and is the main reason I am including stress in this book.

The physiology of stress is fairly complex as it includes a neurological and hormonal response to a physical, mental, psychological or physiological threat or challenge. Even though it is a bit complex, I believe it's helpful to look at all the hormonal and chemical reactions that create the **Stress Response** so that we can more effectively combat it. In the first part of this chapter, I will discuss the most dramatic **Stress Response** called the **Alarm Stage**. This stage of stress engages the emergency system within our body to help survive harrowing situations where we have to "fight or flee." I call this system, initiated within our brain, our internal panic button.

The **Alarm Stage** activates hormones that provide instant energy and mental focus that stimulate many physiological processes. These processes include the acceleration of our heartbeat, shunting blood away from the digestive organs, and the rapid breakdown of glycogen which provides a burst of energy. As this system can quickly deplete energy stores in the body, the **Stress Response** soon moves into the **Adaptation** or **Resistance Stage**, which helps our bodies and minds with prolonged stress. The second section of this chapter will focus on the **Adaptation** or **Resistance Stage**.

The third section will focus on a relatively new player on the scene that profoundly affects our stress level as well as other sources of physiological stress: the **Gut Brain Axis**. In the fourth section, we will look at how stomach problems contribute to stress and, finally, which stress management techniques target each kind of stress.

THE ALARM PHASE

The **Alarm Phase** of the **Stress Response** can be seen as an emergency system that engages our attention and energy so that we can run or fight for our lives. Scientists call this response the **Alarm Phase**. It is probably one of the most important physiological resources within us that allows for the survival of our species, especially when, in the distant past, we were subject to countless threats to our survival. Even though this intense internal mechanism may only rarely be needed in our modern age, this emergency system can still be engaged. The **Alarm Phase** is activated by signals within our brain and deploys many of our nervous and hormonal systems to release **Adrenaline** to key organs, like the heart and lungs, and shunts blood flow and energy away from others, such as our digestive organs. The result is the release of an intense burst of energy where we can run or fight for our lives. The **Alarm Phase** is controlled by two separate and yet almost completely redundant systems. The first system is the **Autonomic Nervous System** (**ANS**) and the second is the **Hypothalmus Pituitary Adrenal Axis** (**HPA**).

Autonomic Nervous System (ANS)

Stress is such a central feature of our biology that it has a dedicated part of our nervous system. The **ANS** initiates the **Stress Response** and when the stress event is over, can return our body to its former state of calm. The **ANS** has nerve branches that travel from the brainstem as well as to areas of the spine, all the major organs, and other important parts of our anatomy including the sinuses. The activation of the **ANS** is an automatic or involuntary process in the body. I use the words automatic or involuntary, because the **Stress Response** often happens whether we consciously direct it or not.

The **ANS** has two main branches:

1. The **Sympathetic Nervous System** (**SNS**); and
2. The **Parasympathetic Nervous System**.

The **SNS** directs the body to produce **Adrenaline** (technically called norepinephrine) for when an immediate surge of energy is required. The **Parasympathetic Nervous System** helps the body produce calming neurochemicals such as **Acetylcholine** and **GABA** which helps to calm the **SNS Adrenaline** response so that the body can rest and digest. Let's look a little more in depth at the **SNS** along with a hormonal system called the **HPA Axis**, which both activate the **Stress Response**. We will examine the **PNS** at the end of this chapter.

The Sympathetic Nervous System (SNS)

The **Sympathetic Nervous System** (SNS) is a set of nerves that create an extensive network travelling to all the major organs and certain areas of the brain. One of the main functions of the **SNS** is to send alarm stress messages to the whole body. Because this response is mediated through the nervous system, the body's response to stress is felt almost immediately. This dedicated nervous system delivers highly stimulating hormones like **Adrenaline** (and to a lesser degree other hormones such as **Cortisol**) that help the body release the energy needed to stay and fight, or to run from a threat. **Adrenaline,** delivered through the nervous system, directly affects many of the organs, especially the heart, elevating the pulse and blood pressure. At the same time, it triggers the shunted blood away from our digestive system. The primary function of the **SNS** is to provide the body with energy to fight or run from a threat.

The HPA Axis: The Second Part of the Panic Button Response

The second phase of the **Alarm Stage** activates a hormonal chain-reaction from the brain to the hypothalamus (the master gland within the brain) to the pituitary gland to the adrenal glands. The adrenal glands are located just above the kidneys. The adrenal glands, then, release a second round of **Adrenaline** (after the initial **SNS** release through the nervous system) that also prepares the body and mind for fight or flight. This hormonal system is called the **Hypothalamus-Pituitary-Adrenal Axis** (**HPA**). Stress is such an important survival response that nature has provided us a backup system that reinforces the **Alarm Stage**, making sure that the panic button is activated and ensuring that these signals arrive at our heart, lungs and adrenal glands, so that we can quickly respond to the stressor.

The **SNS** and the **HPA Axis** both activate the **Alarm System**, and the result is powerful and almost immediate, releasing incredible energy that ensures that we can fight or flee. In modern life, however, this system is rarely fully activated as it is geared toward emergency and life-threatening stress. As many people in modern life no longer face regular life or death situations, very often this panic response is only occasionally engaged, before the **Adaptation of Resistance Stage** kicks in. Modern day stress is usually characterized by stressors we face day-to-day such as pressure at work, problems in our relationships, lack of sleep, or our health. These are more long-term stresses that can create a constant low level of stress often leading to the **Adaptation** or **Resistance** of stress.

Adaptation or Resistance Stress Phase

We all are subject to the surge of adrenalin created by the **SNS** and the **HPA Axis** when in a dangerous or scary situation. When a dangerous or threatening situation continues over a longer period of time, a second stage of the **Stress Response** takes over. This second phase of stress is called the **Adaptation** or **Resistance** Stress Stage, and it is dominated by a second stress hormone called **Cortisol** which helps to sustain the **Stress Response**.

Cortisol is released by the adrenal glands into our bloodstream to ensure that we can sustain more energy and focus to help us to combat an ongoing threat or challenge. The actual function of **Cortisol** is to quickly stimulate the production of glucose by breaking down protein in the liver. This is necessary energy to help maintain the **Stress Response** although at a lower level than provided by **Adrenaline**. **Cortisol** helps us remain vigilant and keeps our bodies in a state of alertness for hours or even days.

Adaptive or **Resistance** Stress, if it lasts for long periods of time, leads to chronic stress and chronic stress can, in turn, lead to burnout and ultimately to exhaustion. If the **Adaptation** or **Resistance** Stage of stress lasts too long, then the protein stores in the liver will become depleted. When that happens, we literally are draining most of our energy stores and, as a result, can feel a deep exhaustion that may last for days or, in extreme situations, weeks or months.

It seems that unpleasant situations have become a feature of our daily life forming a baseline of underlying stress that we all have to cope with. Anytime you feel pressured, overworked, sleep deprived or overwhelmed with life's demands, you are at risk of experiencing the bad effects of chronic stress. Whatever the cause of our stress, the internal mechanisms that release **Cortisol** and the negative effects begin to erode our health and sense of well-being.

The Parasympathetic Nervous System

The **Parasympathetic Nervous System** is a counterbalancing part of the **SNS** that helps the body restore and recover from stress; slowing and undoing many of the stimulating effects of the Sympathetic ramp up of energy. In fact, it is one of the primary ways we can turn off the panic button. The phrase that is commonly associated with the **Parasympathetic**

Nervous System is "rest and digest." More specifically, the purpose of the **Parasympathetic Nervous System** is to restore and rejuvenate the body. Here is a list of all of its functions:

- Conserves energy.
- Increases intestinal motility.
- Slows the heart rate.
- Dilates blood vessels and therefore lowers blood pressure.
- Increases insulin production which helps to control appetite.

There are many things we can do to engage the **Parasympathetic Nervous System**, which we will review in the last section of this chapter, but probably the most obvious **Parasympathetic Nervous System** activity is resting and sleeping. Having a strong **Parasympathetic Nervous System** response is vital to combating stress.

Top-Down Stress Suppresses the Parasympathetic Nervous System and With It, the Immune Response

While the **Parasympathetic Nervous System** is vitally important, it is simply not active during a stress reaction. Even a cold or flu will suppress the **Parasympathetic Nervous System**. This poses a problem for those who wish to lessen the impact and begin healing from a cold or flu viral attack. One of the main problems is caused by the release of **Cortisol** from the **Adaptation** Stage of the **Stress Response**. The reason for this is because **Cortisol** suppresses the **Immune Response**. Moreover, it also diverts the body's resources and energy into maintaining wakefulness while shunting off energy to the digestion. The suppression of the **Immune System** has been corroborated in scientific studies. One example can be found in a meta-study published in 2006 which found that acute and chronic stress significantly suppresses the body's systemic **Immune Response**.[90]

Also included in the long list of bodily processes that are compromised by elevated **Cortisol** is the suppression of insulin which can ultimately increase hunger and interrupt the process of breaking down fat for energy. Moreover, as **Cortisol** is a stimulant, it ends up keying us up which, in turn, can interfere with our sleep. As anyone who has pulled an all-nighter before exams or who has significant jet lag can attest, sleep deprivation can be its own source of stress.

Higher levels of **Cortisol** are also associated with weight gain, osteoporosis, and metabolic disorders such as diabetes as well as the slow erosion of our kidney function. All of these health concerns only increase the effect of stress on our lives and can lead to a vicious cycle where it is difficult to escape the constant drain of stress. This demonstrates the many physiological problems that stress creates simply based on the triggering of **Cortisol** release through the **Adaptive** or **Resistive Stage** of stress.

TOP-DOWN STRESS RESPONSE AND THE MIND

From the description above, we understand a lot about the hormones and neurological and chemical reactions that define a top-down **Stress Response**. The **Stress Response**, directed by the **SNS** and **HPA** as well as the adaptation or resistance stress response, marshalls much of the body's resources and helps us respond when threatened. While the **Stress Response** is, to some degree, an automatic response that we have no control over, scientists have learned that our awareness and mental attitude can help us to become more resilient to stress as well as help to lessen its effects and, in some cases, avoid it altogether.

At its core, the **Stress Response** is an emotional reaction, typically being triggered by fear. For instance, many people are afraid of being negatively affected by a health problem such as cancer or arthritis. This applies not only to the verified negative health problem but also the fear of a future health problems that may or may not occur. The same **Stress Response** can activate the fear of being fired or being betrayed. In fact, the stress experienced by those who have a negative event happen versus the ones who fear that possible future negative events may happen, are virtually identical. They are both driven by our emotions. This same principle can apply to those who are perpetually defensive or angry about being cheated or about the possibility of being cheated. Our stress can serve as a weird coping mechanism that protects us from being negatively surprised in the future.

In this sense, we could say that the **Stress Response** is an odd and often ineffective coping mechanism. But perhaps a more helpful way to look at it is that our minds are prone to worry, to disappointment, to resentment and envy as well as grief and sadness. This especially applies to those people who have grown up in a chaotic or harsh family environment. It also applies to those who have survived a traumatic event such as those experienced by combat soldiers or someone who has been raped or mugged. Whatever the reason, many of us need support to help them put things into perspective or simply receive the support of a caring person who provides a non-judgemental space to help us sort out our feelings.

This is why, counseling or even the listening ear of a friend, can be invaluable in our quest to unravel the complexity of our stress reactions, including our family history and the difficulties we have faced in our life. However we choose to explore and help heal from our stress, we must keep in mind that stress is often fed by our internal dialogue and thought processes regarding our challenges. For this reason, meditation, prayer and other stress relieving activities can specifically help to quiet the mind and thereby help us to refocus our attention.

In fact, when we slow down and stop ruminating, often much of the stress falls away. Also, to express our feelings and put them into the context of our life experience, can often help us to gain perspective and begin a process of healing. This can help us to feel happier and less subject to the many ups and downs of life. Feelings can have many layers and many people find that they need help in becoming aware of and understanding their feelings on a deeper level.

In the final section, I will provide helpful solutions to dealing with this kind of emotional stress. To those who explore this avenue of healing, it is often a slow and challenging process but can provide real, lasting relief from much of the effects of stress. The next section will explore the **Gut Brain Axis**, which is perhaps the most hidden and insidious form of stress and demonstrates why stress can affect us even if we have sufficient control over our reactions to the difficulties of work and family.

THE GUT BRAIN AXIS

Understanding and coping with stress has been the subject of considerable research since the discovery by physiologist Dr. Hans Selye that stress was a real physiological event with real, measurable effects. Dr. Selye discovered the physiological basis of stress in 1936 and continued to study it throughout his lifetime. His scientific work elaborated on the complex interactions of the **Autonomic Nervous System** and its component parts, the **Sympathetic** and **Parasympathetic Nervous Systems**, creating the initial framework that defined and helped scientists understand stress.

Selye's work on stress has provided a comprehensive understanding of the top-down **Stress Response**. However, recent developments in research have revealed a much more complex biological underpinning to stress. At the center of this new understanding is the realization that inflammation centered in the network of nerves interwoven in the gut, called the **Enteric Nervous System (ENS)**[91] or the **Gut Microbiome** (the bacterial lining of the intestines), together with the **Autonomic Nervous System**, generate the **Stress Response**. Together, these biological systems create a dynamic system in our body which has profound effects on our stress levels. The **ENS** and the **Autonomic Nervous System**, along with the **Gut Microbiome** are collectively called the **Gut Brain Axis**. This new understanding is now referred to as a bottom-up activation of the **Stress Response.**[92] As the **Gut Brain Axis** is an overarching term that covers three major systems, we should discuss them individually so we may understand how they interact and trigger a **Stress Response**.

STRESS FROM THE BOTTOM UP

Looking at stress from the bottom-up means we will now look at how problems with digestion strongly impact our stress. Bottom-up stress is almost always created by gut inflammation problems such as **GERD** (commonly known as heartburn) or **Irritable Bowel Syndrome**. We will begin our discussion with the **ENS** as a key part of the **Gut-Brain Axis**.

The ENS and the Gut Brain Axis

The **ENS** (also called the **Second Brain**[93]) is composed of approximately 200 to 500 million neurons, which is more neurons than the spinal cord, interwoven into the tissues of the gut. These neurons sense the state of the digestive organs as well as that of other organs such as the stomach and heart, and direct much of the digestive process. The **ENS** communicates with the brain primarily through the **Vagus Nerve** which travels from the brainstem through the back of the neck into the chest, before continuing down to the stomach and abdominal area. This unique nerve serves as a conduit for information that flows from the **ENS** to the brain (**CNS**). The **Vagus Nerve**, in addition to being a primary neurological connection of the **Gut-Brain Axis**, is also a key component of the **Parasympathetic Nervous System**, delivering a significant amount of Neurotransmitters associated with the rest and digest function of this part of the **Autonomic Nervous System**.

THE VAGUS NERVE'S EFFECT ON STRESS

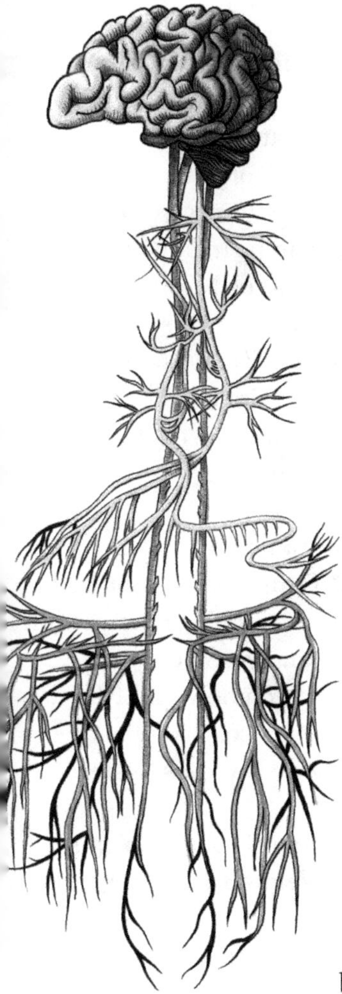

The **Vagus Nerve** is currently a hot topic in medicine but has not always enjoyed the limelight of the scientific world. Every medical student studies this nerve as the main branch of the **Parasympathetic Nervous System**, and as an important counter measure to the **Sympathetic Nervous System**. It was Dr. Michael Gershon who discovered the **Vagus Nerve**'s critical role as the chief method with which the **ENS** communicates with the brain. His groundbreaking work helped to bring attention to the **ENS** as well as the **Vagus Nerve**, and ultimately how the **Gut Brain Axis** controls bottom-up stress.

Based on the discoveries of Dr. Gershon and many others, we now know that gut inflammation interferes with **ENS** and **Vagus Nerve** function. The impact on the **Vagus Nerve** function is particularly problematic because the **Vagus Nerve** comprises 75% of the Parasympathetic System in the body. When the gut is inflamed, the **Vagus Nerve**'s function becomes compromised. When this happens, it is called **Low Vagal Tone. Low Vagal Tone** is a surprisingly troublesome problem as it partially blocks the information and neurochemicals that should be transmitted to the brain. Moreover, as **Vagal Tone** is critical for the **Parasympathetic Nervous System** to fully function, this creates a significant imbalance in our **Stress Response**. In fact, the **Vagus Nerve** is the center of the bottom-up **Stress Response** and the reason why **GERD, Silent Reflux, Gut Microbiome** problems and what I call **Temporary Silent Reflux** (from an **ENS** viral cold or flu) can all amp up our stress.

In the next two sections, I will review how these types of digestive problems interfere with our **Vagus Nerve** function and create bottom-up stress.

GERD, STRESS AND INFLAMMATION

GERD (commonly called heartburn) and **Silent Reflux** (a milder version of **GERD**) both are inflammatory diseases that affect millions of people. These two stomach problems are centered in the **ENS Zone** and have a substantial impact on the **Gut-Brain Axis**. **GERD** generates dramatic symptoms such as acid reflux and heartburn. These symptoms are actually caused by an inflammatory process at the junction of the stomach or **Lower Esophageal Sphincter** which, in turn, causes the **ENS** to be inflamed. All this inflammation interferes with the ability of the **Vagus Nerve** to transmit Parasympathetic chemicals such as **Acetylcholine**. This shunting of **Acetylcholine** is, in fact, a defining characteristic of **Low Vagal Tone**.[94] In other words, **GERD** or **Silent Reflux** effectively disable a significant part of the **Parasympathetic Nervous System**. This makes it far more challenging for people suffering from these conditions to rest, relax and digest.

With this new understanding of bottom-up stress, we can gain a fuller perspective of how an **ENS** Viral Cold can generate **Temporary Silent Reflux** symptoms and not only cause a sore throat, but also create **ENS** inflammation and **Low Vagal Tone**. As an **ENS** Viral Cold shares many of the same symptoms that are found in **Silent Reflux**, light is shed on how an **ENS** Viral Cold can generate colds symptoms and explain why colds and flus feel stressful, causing interference with the **Parasympathetic Nervous System**.

There is yet another bottom-up issue that can create significant problems for the **Gut-Brain Axis** as well as contribute to **Low Vagus Tone**. This is the **Gut Microbiome**. In the last few years, literally hundreds of new research papers have been slowly unraveling the mysteries of the vast bacterial colony that inhabits our intestines. In the next seven sections, we'll explore some highlights of this system and how it affects bottom-up stress.

THE GUT MICROBIOME AND STRESS

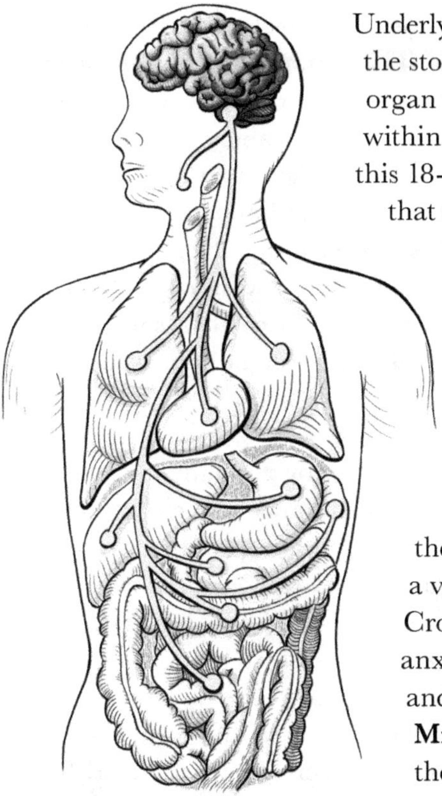

Underlying the **ENS** are several organs such as the stomach, liver and kidneys. The dominant organ that occupies the majority of the space within the abdomen is the intestines. Within this 18-foot organ is a vast bacterial colony that forms its lining. This living lining, composed almost entirely of bacteria, is called the **Gut Microbiome**. This colony of trillions of bacteria helps our intestines and our body absorb and produce nutrients which are vital for our sustained energy and vitality. In the last 20 years, many studies have been published that link the condition of the **Gut Microbiome** with a variety of health conditions including Crohn's Disease, Lupus, depression and anxiety, fibromyalgia, rheumatoid arthritis, and headaches. More importantly, the **Gut Microbiome** is now emerging as a one of the leading causes of digestive problems such as **Irritable Bowel Syndrome.**[95]

The Gut Microbiome Has an Exaggerated Stress Response

Formative research is emerging showing the significance of a healthy **Gut Microbiome** on reducing stress. One recent study showed that mice with no gut bacteria have an exaggerated response to stress.[96] That exaggerated **Stress Response** was corrected, in the same study, by administering probiotics.[97] One journal states that "(a)ccumulating evidence lends support to the view that pro-inflammatory **cytokines** have a role in hyperactivation of the **HPA Axis**."[98] One leading theory that explains why **Gut Microbiome** imbalances can lead to stress is **Leaky Gut Syndrome**. Below, the implications of **Leaky Gut Syndrome** on bottom-up stress will be discussed.

Gut Microbiome and Leaky Gut

Leaky Gut Syndrome is a **Gut Microbiome** problem caused when unhealthy bacteria dominates the **Gut Microbiome**. These unhealthy bacteria, called **Endotoxins**, increase gut inflammation and gut permeability which is often referred to as **Leaky Gut Syndrome**. Intestinal permeability is now a well-established phenomenon where **Endotoxins** and other intestinal by-products "leak" through the intestinal wall. All this leaking of **Endotoxins** and other undigested food, initiates an **Immune Response** causing the gut to become inflamed. This increased inflammation also interferes with **Vagus Nerve** function and leads to **Low Vagal Tone**. **Low Vagal Tone** always interferes with the **Vagus Nerve**'s ability to provide the **Parasympathetic Nervous System**'s rest and digestive function.

Low Vagal Tone not only causes bottom-up stress by disabling the **Parasympathetic Nervous System** but has been shown to increase the **Innate Immune Cell** response creating an exaggerated pro-inflammatory response.[99,100] With this exaggerated inflammatory response, the body is not able to function normally. For instance, without the ability to rest and digest, our ability to absorb nutrients is compromised leading to lower energy. Also, resources that we need for being active and alert are redirected to the exaggerated **Immune Response**. This can create a negative feedback loop where the heightened inflammatory environment creates lower **Vagal Tone**, which in turn further escalates gut inflammation. This downward spiral of inflammation progressively increasing **Low Vagal Tone**, creates further dysfunction of the **ENS** and the **Parasympathetic Nervous System**.[101] This chain reaction of disabling the **Vagus Nerve** and the **Parasympathetic Nervous System** shows how problematic bottom-up stress can be.

In the last section, we will look at natural solutions to reverse these problems and help to restore the **Gut Brain Axis** and **Vagal Tone** to normal function. Before we look at solutions, let us examine two more problems that result from bottom-up stressors. These are mood problems and sleep problems.

Mood and Our Microbiome

New research now shows the **Gut Microbiome** is intimately connected to our mood. In fact, it is now well-established that people with unhealthy bacteria in their **Gut Microbiome** are more susceptible to mood disorders such as depression and anxiety.[102,103,104] New discoveries about the **Gut Microbiome** show that a healthy **Gut Microbiome** creates hormones that support happiness; while an unhealthy **Gut Microbiome** interferes with the production of these hormones. In fact, **Gut Microbiome** produces 95% of the **Serotonin** (the happiness hormone) and 50% of the **Dopamine** (the hormone primarily associated with motivation) along with many other hormones that influence our mental health.[05]

Anyone who has had to combat depression and/or anxiety can attest that these conditions can be very isolating, frustrating and quite stressful while, at the same time, sapping motivation to take steps to manage these stressors. Much more research is needed in this area to fully understand this relationship between the **Gut Microbiome** and mood. However, there are cutting edge nutrition protocols that are showing some success with patients with depression or anxiety that focus on improving the balance of bacteria within the **Gut Microbiome**. I will review some of the basics around this protocol as well as other measures to lessen **Low Vagal Tone** in the last section of this book.

Insomnia and Gut Brain Axis

Sleep disorders are now pervasive in America, and considered to be a significant health-related problem affecting one in three adults.[106] The scale of the problem can be clearly seen in the sheer number of available sleep medications, with sales rising over $5 billion a year or more. Insomnia is a complex problem but much of the blame for this problem can be placed on the high levels of stress in our society. Given that stress is a big part of the issue, many patients find little relief through conventional therapies. In fact, many patients are surprised just how inadequate modern medicine is in solving this significant health challenge, finding themselves taking medications that only partially solve the dilemma and are usually accompanied by a whole host of unpleasant side effects.

New answers are emerging centered around inflammatory gut problems including the inflammation generated by **GERD** and **Silent Reflux**, as well as an unhealthy **Gut Microbiome**. Clearly, all these complications lead to **Low Vagal Tone** and thereby activate a bottom-up **Stress Response**. All of these conditions lead to a disabling of the **Parasympathetic Nervous System**, making it much more difficult for people with this problem to fully relax and sleep. This newer perspective is reflected in a recent study where **Low Vagal Tone** was implicated in poor sleep.[107]

Also, medical researchers now know that people who have trouble falling or staying asleep have higher blood markers for inflammation.[108] Paradoxically, as we will see in one of the final sections of this book, one of the best natural means of lessening stress is sleep which naturally restores **Vagal Tone**.

For most people, sleep is not an optional activity. We know that sleep stimulates the **Parasympathetic Nervous System** which is a built-in counter-measure for the **Adrenaline/Cortisol**-based **Stress Response**. Sleep is therefore a critically important resource that we need to be healthy.

STRESS FROM THE TOP DOWN OR BOTTOM UP

One of the most important puzzles we must solve in our quest to be healthy while reducing our stress is to determine whether it is top-down or bottom-up stress. Many of my patients have found a natural approach utilizing strategies to heal the **Gut-Brain Axis**, helping them deal with their stress as well as their sleep problems. Of course, top-down stress will ultimately create bottom-up stress and bottom-up stress often leads to top-down stressors as well. You should examine all stress-management solutions with this in mind. I will provide some basic holistic suggestions for both these problems in the final section of the chapter. This especially applies to anyone who is interested in reducing the frequency of their colds and flus as those who get less sleep tend to be more vulnerable to becoming sick.[109]

Maintaining a Healthy Gut Microbiome

Much can be said about the ecological balance of the **Gut Microbiome** which serves as a foundation of healthy digestion and overall health. The **Gut Microbiome** impacts our stress when the balance of good and unhealthy bacteria of the **Gut Microbiome** is disrupted.

Fostering education around the **Gut Microbiome** has been one of the main jobs within my practice. The information I and many other qualified healthcare professionals offer can have a life-changing impact on a patient's overall health and stress level. One of the most important things that I communicate around maintaining a healthy **Gut Microbiome** is drawing awareness to the many prescribed or over-the-counter medications that negatively affect it.

Given this connection between a healthy **Gut Microbiome** and stress, it is essential to learn more about how to maintain a healthy bacterial balance in the intestine. One of the most important ways of maintaining a healthy **Gut Microbiome** is to avoid, or at least limit, taking certain medications.

The most detrimental prescription medications to the **Gut Microbiome** are antibiotics. Afterall, antibiotics are usually taken orally, and this medicine enters eventually into the intestines which houses the trillions of bacteria that constitute the **Gut Microbiome**. Antibiotics kill the bad bacteria as well as the good bacteria. One of my functions as a healthcare provider is to find, when possible, an alternative to antibiotics. I have developed counter-measures that patients can take to protect their **Gut Microbiome** if they must take a regiment of antibiotics. I will review these in the last section.

Other medications that negatively affect the **Gut Microbiome** include steroids,[110] hormones,[111] chemotherapy drugs,[112] and NSAIDS (common painkillers/anti-inflammatories).[113] All of these medications can be life-saving or help relieve pain, so patients should heed their doctor's advice. However, sometimes these medicines can be reduced or even replaced with a more natural alternative herbal medicine or treatment such as acupuncture. Moreover, I found that many physicians were willing to postpone their prescription and allow me to prescribe an herb or supplement to see if that worked first. Suffice to say, these decisions are often dependent on open communication and having a good rapport with your alternative and conventional health practitioners. I will review alternatives to some of these medications in the final section of this chapter.

Health Check

DO I HAVE LOW VAGAL NERVE TONE?

Patients often come to me feeling stressed, looking for a healthy way to feel better. Often, I find that they have a **Gut Brain Axis** problem. I look at these kinds of problems first, in terms of the severity of their symptoms. Do they have a mild, moderate or extreme problem? I then try to determine if they have a stomach problem such as **GERD**, **Silent Reflux** or a **Gut Microbiome** issue. Occasionally, they may have more than one of these problems. Here are some of the criteria I use to assess if their problem is bottom-up stress. Readers should go through this list and see if any of these symptoms apply. This should help to determine if your stress is primarily Top-Down or Bottom-Up. Of course, many people suffer from both Top-Down and Bottom-Up stress. If that is the case, start with treating Bottom-Up stress and monitor the results.

Silent Reflux Symptoms (check all that apply):

- ❏ I wake up with a sore throat
- ❏ I'm tired after eating acidic food like tomatoes, tomato sauce or citrus or a coffee beverage
- ❏ My ears, palate or the back of my throat are often itchy
- ❏ I have intermittent chest pressure
- ❏ I catch colds frequently that always start with a sore throat
- ❏ Stress management is challenging for me
- ❏ I often have problems swallowing

Mild GERD

- ❏ I have mild burning in my throat frequently
- ❏ The burning gets a bit worse after eating acidic food like tomatoes, tomato sauce or citrus or a beverage like coffee
- ❏ I have mild heartburn
- ❏ I can't lie flat without getting some heartburn or mild burning in the throat
- ❏ I occasionally burp up acid

Moderate GERD

- ❏ I have mild to moderate burning in my throat or heartburn
- ❏ I sometimes wake with significant burning in my chest or throat
- ❏ I must go to the doctor as this problem affects my ability to sleep or eat
- ❏ I need medications such as Proton Pump inhibitors to control these problems
- ❏ I need to avoid all acidic foods or drink or else I suffer from GERD symptoms

Severe GERD

- ❑ I have constant intense burning in my throat or chest
- ❑ I need to go to the emergency room frequently for this burning in my throat
- ❑ I can have an emergency situation if I eat or drink acidic food
- ❑ I am on two or more Proton Pump Inhibitors

Mild Gut Microbiome Problem

- ❑ I have gas or bloating
- ❑ I have occasional loose stools or constipation
- ❑ I always get more gassy after eating anything with sugar and starches

Moderate Gut Microbiome Problem

- ❑ I have frequent diarrhea or loose stools (up to 5 times a day)
- ❑ I have chronic constipation and have bowel movements every 1 to 3 days
- ❑ I have alternating diarrhea and constipation
- ❑ I have been diagnosed with Irritable Bowel Syndrome or Fibromyalgia
- ❑ I have restless sleep
- ❑ I have trouble staying still and fidget frequently when sitting or trying to sleep
- ❑ I have some brain fog and have trouble concentrating
- ❑ I have some abdominal pain
- ❑ There is occasionally blood in my stool
- ❑ I have frequent frontal headaches (headaches in and around the forehead and eyes)
- ❑ I feel better from exercise
- ❑ I feel better from fasting or going on a very restricted low carb, no sugar diet
- ❑ I am frequently stressed out
- ❑ I catch colds or the flu extremely easily

Extreme Gut Microbiome Problem

- ❑ I have severe diarrhea 6 to 20 times a day
- ❑ I have chronic constipation and have bowel movements every 4 to 8 days
- ❑ There is often bleeding accompanying my stool
- ❑ I have been to the hospital for an impaction issue
- ❑ I have alternating diarrhea and constipation all day, every day
- ❑ I have been diagnosed with Irritable Bowel Syndrome or an Irritable Bowel Disease like Crohn's Disease or another auto-immune disease such as Lupus or Rheumatoid Arthritis

- ❑ I have very restless sleep and have trouble getting much sleep at all
- ❑ I can have severe abdominal pain and have been to the hospital for emergency pain relief
- ❑ I can't function in a normal way in life and probably can't work or go out with friends
- ❑ I am always extremely stressed out
- ❑ I catch colds or the flu extremely easily

NOTE: If you have checked two or more items on this list, refer to the end of this chapter for treatment recommendations.

RESULT: ______________________________

WHY CATCHING A COLD FEELS STRESSFUL

It's taken me many years to put the whole picture together, but I now know that we are fighting two battles when we have a cold or flu. One battle is from fighting off the viral infection and the other is battling the bottom-up stress associated with the inflammation of a virally-infected **ENS**. Even those without a stomach or **Gut Microbiome** problem, will temporarily suffer from **ENS** inflammation and **Temporary Silent Reflux** caused by a cold or flu virus, and therefore will experience stress. This means that cold sufferers are in double jeopardy as rising levels of cortisone gradually suppress the **Immune Response** while **Low Vagal Tone** progressively disables the **Parasympathetic Nervous System** and creates an exaggerated pro-inflammatory **Immune Response** (primarily stimulating **Macrophages**).

An **ENS** cold has symptoms caused by the blending of **Immune Response** reactions, like **Temporary Silent Reflux** as well as some level of **Stress Response.** When we look at what causes the symptoms of a cold, we can see that fever and abdominal heat are caused by the **Immune System** attacking the viral infection. **Temporary Silent Reflux** is caused by the inflammation at the **Lower Esophageal Sphincter**, resulting in a sore throat as well as the symptoms of the **Stress Response**, which may include a knot in the stomach, a tight neck, and/or sinus congestion. **Low Vagal Tone** contributes to the stressful feeling of a cold or flu and results in fatigue, poor sleep, and a dull thinking process from a disabled **Parasympathetic Nervous System**.

Low mood associated with the cold could be the result of a combination of an unhealthy **Gut Microbiome** made worse by **Low Vagal Tone**. For those who are unaware of holistic measures, their most effective treatment strategy when combating the onset of a cold is to rest, thereby stimulating the **Parasympathetic Nervous System**, and wait for their **Immune Response** to gather sufficient numbers to fight the virus off.

However, for those who have access to a holistic practitioner, receiving acupuncture, massage, or gentle Osteopathic manual therapy can also reduce the **Stress Response** and help to restore blood flow to the digestive organs and the **ENS**, in turn increasing **Vagal Tone** and reducing the release of **Cortisol**. These measures alone can help to speed the progress of a common cold or flu while also helping to reduce the symptoms.

Now that we have a more comprehensive view of stress and what stresses us out, we can focus on how to combat our stress. The first natural healing strategy is to activate the **PNS**.

WAYS TO REDUCE OUR STRESS

With so many sources of stress triggering the **SNS**, **HPA** and **Adaptive** or Resistive **Stress Response**, as well as **Low Vagal Tone**, stomach, and **Gut Microbiome** issues, it's little wonder that so many of us struggle to successfully manage our stress, even as we realize how profoundly it effects our health and how much it's heightens our risk of catching colds and flus. In this section, I will review a selection of stress management tools. First, I should say, there are no drugs that I am aware of that are designed specifically to reduce your stress. Even herbs have limited benefits to those who are stressed for long periods of time. However, there are proven strategies to help us effectively manage our stress and unravel the vicious cycle that depletes our energies and compromises our **Immune Response** to colds and flus.

Reducing the Impact of the Sympathetic Nervous System

Several strategies can be employed to reduce stress or at least the impact of stress on our lives. Next, we will look at strategies to help the body get rid of the build-up of stress hormones that are the inevitable result of a revved up **Sympathetic Nervous System**.

Aerobic Exercise

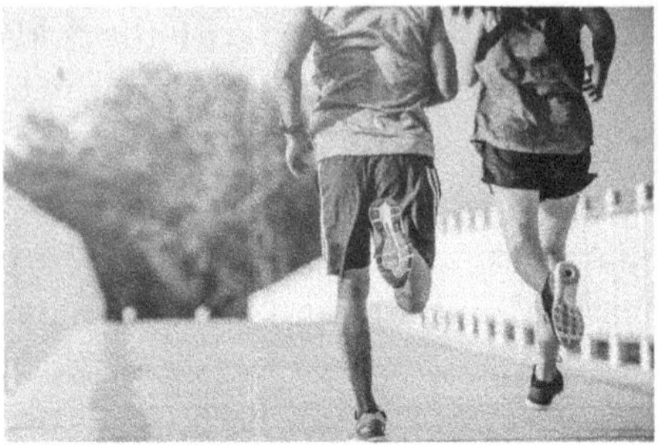

Aerobic exercise can be an effective way for the body to rid itself of all the hormones associated with stress. With the release of **Adrenaline** and **Cortisol**, the body remains in a constant state of alert and, until the hormones are eventually reabsorbed, it is very hard to fully relax. Exercise speeds up this process by increasing blood flow and amping up the body's metabolism. Thirty minutes or more of aerobic exercise appears to be helpful for long-term stress relief. However, it is now known that by itself, aerobic exercise also suppresses the **Parasympathetic Nervous System**, which is vital to lowering our stress.[114] We must learn techniques that also stimulate the **Parasympathetic Nervous System** in concert with aerobic exercise to truly effectively reduce stress.

Obviously, aerobic exercise can only be practiced when we are well. If you become ill with a cold, aerobic exercise is depleting and all too often, in the process of cooling down from a workout, a cold sufferer will find that they activate more blood flow and in doing so increase the **Innate Immune Response**, which can elevate fever and increase other symptoms.[115] Therefore, aerobic exercise is a prevention measure to help us lower our stress when we're healthy rather than something to help overcome a cold.

Herbal Teas

One of the most important strategies that may be employed to alleviate stress is drinking herbal tea. Certain herbs have been identified as helpful in assisting the body cope with higher levels of stress. These herbs are categorized as **Adaptog**ens and have been the focus of a number of studies that validate their usefulness in helping people become more resilient to the effects of stress. Herbs such as Siberian Ginseng, Rhodiola, and Ashwagandha have significant research backing their use.[116,117,118] While these are usually not a long-term solution for stress, they are ideal when we need an emergency boost to our energy without side effects, especially when we're sleep deprived, working long hours or experiencing another very stressful event.

Also, herbs that help the body combat the cold, such as Shinus Molle and Andrographis, have some benefit. I will review sources and dosages in the next sections of this chapter. There are many, many herbs that are utilized in treating the common cold, but, after being in practice for 27 years, the herbs on this list are my top picks.

Herbs and Supplements that Help to Reduce Inflammation in the Stomach and ENS

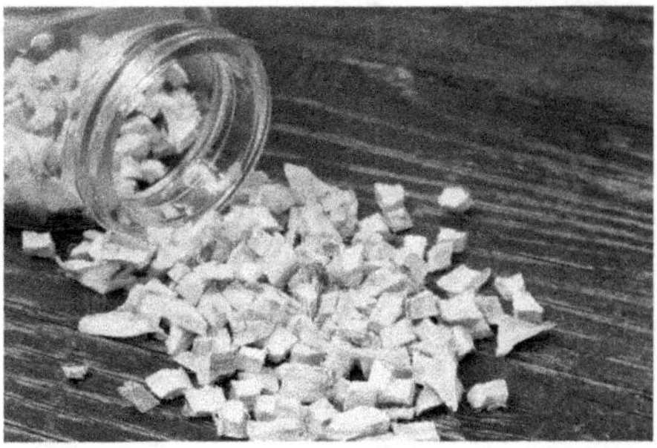

The main herbs that I recommend for reducing the inflammation in the **ENS** are Omega-3 fish oil, Slippery Elm, and Marshmallow Root. Omega-3 fish oil is a systemic anti-inflammatory while the other two are primarily for the stomach, although they can help to soothe a sore throat. If you have a higher fever or severe sore throat, I recommend that you refer to protocols suggested in the Immune Chapter before trying these herbs. After the fever has subsided, Slippery Elm and/or Marshmallow Root can really help to lessen **Temporary Silent Reflux** symptoms. This also applies to fish oil which usually only helps after the intense symptoms of a cold or flu have subsided. All of these remedies should help to lessen **Lower Esophageal Sphincter** inflammation and help to restore the **Parasympathetic Nervous System**.

Gut Microbiome Support

The main supplement for the **Gut Microbiome** is probiotics. Probiotics should also be considered only after the fever has broken and the symptoms are less intense. Probiotics will often help to lessen the impact of **Low Vagal Tone**. I recommend two pills every twelve hours of a high-quality probiotic. Patients with **Gut Microbiome** issues should also avoid any food with sugar and high carbohydrate foods such as bread or pasta. For moderate to severe cases, patients should seek the guidance of a qualified healthcare provider who specializes in **Gut Microbiome** problems.

Taking bitter herbs is important to help regulate **Gut Microbiome** issues as it will help to create an environment conducive to beneficial bacteria. I discuss dosage and timing at length in the *Chapter 5, Eliminating Your Cough by Clearing Out Clutter.*

Supporting the Parasympathetic Nervous System

Rest

The most basic method to stimulate the **Parasympathetic Nervous System** is rest. As an example, many students going through finals, often return home and sleep for long periods of time. This is their way of stimulating the **Parasympathetic Nervous System** and restoring balance to the **Autonomic Nervous System**. Of course, as our responsibilities increase, long periods of rest are a luxury most people cannot afford. It is one of the main reasons people relish their vacations as they can have more time to rest and recover from the unrelenting stress in their lives. It is also a slow but effective strategy to combat a cold.

Yoga, Tai Chi, Chi Gong

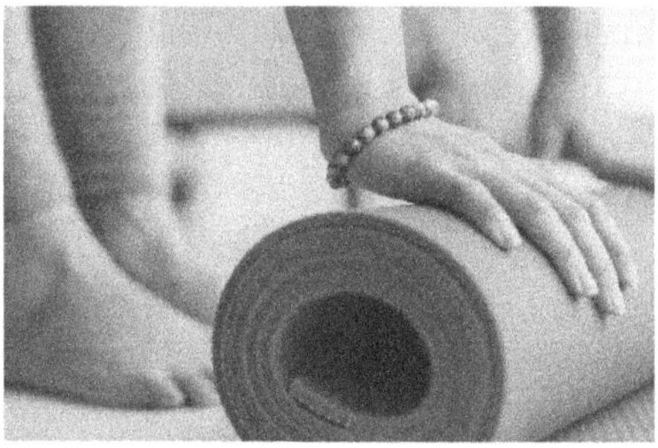

Any exercise program that is deeply relaxing will stimulate the **Parasympathetic Nervous System**. These activities usually focus on slow, conscious movements, coordinating breath and movement together. I personally feel that these exercises help us in many ways. For instance, they help us to slow down, breathe more deeply, and focus in a relaxed way. This is helpful to those who wish to address their stress with real exercise that encourages good posture and letting go of top-down stressors of the day. Over time, these practices can train our bodies and minds so that we are more relaxed when performing other activities like driving to work or typing on a computer. Because these exercises encourage deep breathing and movements that bring more blood flow to the core, they also help with reducing **Sympathetic Nervous System** hormones like **Adrenaline** and **Cortisol** while helping the body to heal from **Low Vagal Tone**.

For anyone who is unfamiliar with yoga, Tai Chi or Qigong, it is important to find a teacher that helps you learn these more refined forms of exercise. For many, going to a favored teacher each week can serve as a foundation for ongoing stress-management and a structured, safe and rewarding way to address stress. It is not for nothing that yoga has grown in popularity in the

U.S. In fact, a recent study has shown that people doing "yoga has grown by over 50% in the last four years to over 36 million as of 2016, up from 20.4 million in 2012. In addition, nine out of 10 Americans have heard of yoga, one in three Americans has tried yoga at least once, and more than 15% of Americans have done yoga in the last 6 months".[119,120]

Meditation and Guided Relaxation

Meditation and Guided Relaxation both help us to deeply relax and experience stress reduction and improvement of mood.[121] There are scores of studies that highlight the stress-reducing benefits of yoga in the workplace as a way of reducing burn out, which is code for stress.[122] One specific programs that have been researched in the medical field include Mindfulness Meditation. Meditation, in order to be effective, must be practiced for at least 15 minutes a day for many months.

Acupuncture

Several studies show that acupuncture provides temporary **Vagal Nerve** stimulation and helps to down-regulate the overactive **Immune Response** while increasing the **Parasympathetic Nervous System** activity.[123] While these results are temporary, it can provide valuable assistance in the process of fighting a cold by eliminating an exaggerated pro-inflammatory response to the virus while helping a patient to reduce the stress associated with a cold. Research is emerging that verifies that acupuncture also helps to make the body more resilient to stress. The was demonstrated by observing certain hormones including cortisone elevation. The study confirmed that 10 acupuncture treatments helped long term to reduce the release of these hormones long term.[124] You should feel the positive effects of Acupuncture even with a single treatment. If you have tried it without success, it means you should look for a more skilled practitioner.

Osteopathic Manual Therapy

A highly-trained Osteopathic Physician can often help to engage the **Parasympathetic Nervous System** through the gentle manipulation of the cranial bones as well as the spine. Treating the **ANS** is a specialty of Osteopathy which not only helps to calm the **Stress Response** but also helps to recruit blood flow and the body's resources against the virus. The result can often speed the course of a cold while simultaneously calming the **Stress Response**. Typically, patients report significant relief from just a few treatments.

Deep Breathing

Taking slow, deep breaths throughout our day helps us to release the diaphragm, which is the muscle right behind the stress knot in our stomachs. Most of us don't realize that when we're stressed we tend to hold our breath and breathe more shallowly. Deep breathing overrides this tendency and simultaneously triggers a **Parasympathetic Nervous System** response.[125]

Psychotherapy

Top-down stress is often complex and we often unwittingly contribute to our own stress by getting involved in relationships that lack true intimacy or empathy. Often, many people make poor choices due to poor communication skills or blind spots where they lack understanding of how to address and unravel stress. Others find themselves in situations that elicit situational stress, such as the loss of a loved one or a betrayal by a loved one. In these and other situations, often therapy offers ways for us to process our feelings, judgments, and attitudes so that we can navigate our lives without creating more stress for ourselves.

There are many therapists who can offer true support and guidance as we learn to make changes and explore our inner workings. Therapists tend to specialize in different aspects of mental health, so I encourage anyone who wishes to engage a therapist, to do a phone interview with several before selecting one . The result can be rewarding and help to eliminate some of the stress that interferes with mental and emotional well-being.

For those who wish for an alternative to traditional psychotherapy, there are many non-traditional forms of individual and group therapy that work to help us to experience deep emotional transformation. Many of these alternative therapies are based on the work of Carl Jung, the principle student of Freud. Examples of these alternative therapies include Shadow Work, Mankind Project, Women Within, and Hakomi therapy. The training for these therapies is extensive so I encourage anyone who explores them to make sure that their therapist is certified or has extensive experience. Mankind Project and Women Within are intensive weekend workshops that are also rewarding.

Massage Therapy

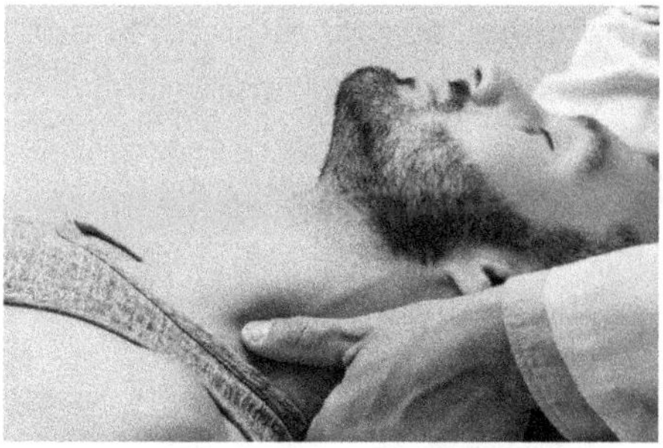

For some, not all, massage therapy offers a relaxing, nurturing experience that de-stresses the body. There are many types of massage and it's hard to make a blanket recommendation on which type of massage will help de-stress your body. For instance, deep tissue massage is favored by some and considered painful and uncomfortable by others. The same applies to Swedish, Shiatsu, and Triggerpoint. These massage techniques are all focused more on deep sustained pressure. For those who prefer a lighter touch, there are several styles that will appeal more to you such as Polarity Therapy, Healing Touch, and Reiki Therapy.

Massage is something I consider an adjunct therapy that can enhance and deepen your stress management. However, in my opinion, massage works more deeply and completely if you exercise and have a guided relaxation or meditation practice.

Herbal Therapy

The main oral herb protocol is bitter herbs which are reviewed in *Chapter 5, Eliminating Your Cough by Clearing Out Clutter.* The main topical herbal therapy for supporting the **Parasympathetic Nervous System** in my clinic is Shinus Molle. This herb has research that indicates it has antibiotic and antifungal properties., My interest in this herb is in its anti-inflammatory and sedation properties.[126,127] There is mounting evidence that this has potent anti-inflammatory effects even when applied topically.[128,129,130] This South American herb, which is traditionally used to treat the common cold, has potent essential oils that appear to have an almost immediate positive effect on **Low Vagal Tone**, reducing abdominal fever and helping to reduce the bottom-up **Stress Response**.

As the active ingredients in Schinus Molle are all essential oils, Shinus Molle tea is not helpful as essential oils evaporate when exposed to boiling water. I make an alcohol-water percolation that extracts the key essential oils and apply this topically on the epigastric area every 3 to 4 hours, until the abdominal fever is resolved. Shinus Molle essential oil is also now sufficiently popular to be sold commercially.

While topical Shinus Molle is helpful to increase **Vagal Tone** by itself, it is not sufficient to combat a serious cold or flu. Most patients will find that medicinal mushrooms, explained in depth in the **Immune System** chapter, must also be used to fully treat an **ENS** viral cold or flu infection.

STRESS MANAGEMENT IS A LIFESTYLE

The therapies list above are life-altering and should be considered as a way to manage our stress. Hopefully, people reading this won't conclude that they should start a yoga or tai chi class only when they're sick! I am a big fan of exercise, even if you have a fabulous Acupuncturist, Osteopath or Massage Therapist. Exercise offers a unique way to increase our stress resilience and helps to naturally help to destress the body and mind. It is important to seek out a teacher (whether it's yoga or whatever other form of exercise you chose) that inspires you and helps you to find a deeper sense of fulfillment and inner calm while promoting a more consistent sense of well-being.

Managing our stress is the first step into a completely different life where we find a deeper sense of ourselves and a way to successfully combat the daily pressures and challenges of stress.

The next section will discuss coughs in depth, which will provide additional informaiton and treatment options for **Low Vagal Tone**.

CHAPTER 5
Eliminating Your Cough by Clearing Out Clutter: A Plan for Detoxification to Restore the Function of Your Mucosal Immune Response

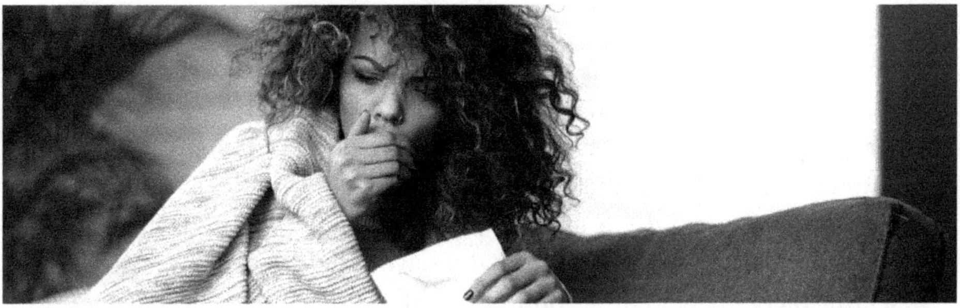

This chapter provides holistic strategies to treat coughs successfully. There are three different types of coughs outlined in this chapter, each requiring a different holistic therapy. Treating coughs with a foundational understanding of **ENS colds** has been quite useful and has helped me to understand the mechanisms of coughs. Doctors and researchers are also beginning to investigate the relationship between stomach problems such as **GERD** to chronic coughs.[131] Just like sore throats, most coughs can be related to the **Silent Reflux** symptoms that we reviewed in the *Chapter 2, Second Brain* as well as the *Chapter 4, The Body's Secret Regulator.* I categorize coughs into three types:

1. Intense gagging coughs at the onset of a cold.
2. Dry coughs from a "tickle" feeling in the throat.
3. Coughs from the irritation of postnasal drip.

GAGGING COUGH

The first type of cough, intense gagging coughs, are almost always associated with severe viral flu. A person with this cough typically coughs uncontrollably, is chilled, and quite miserable. These symptoms are typical of a flu-related cough that requires frequent dosing of herbal medicine as it indicates that the viral infection is quite active. I recommend 2,000 to 3,000 milligrams of medicinal mushrooms every hour for up to 8 hours until the chill and cough subside. Also, applying 10 to 20 drops of Brazilian Peppertree (Schinus Molle) over the epigastric area (just below the rib cage) on the upper abdomen can give excellent temporary relief.

TICKLE OR DRY COUGH

For many, a tickle cough tends to come as an end-stage of the cold. These patients complain of a persistent cough due to a "tickle" or irritation in the throat. I have found that this is primarily due to the aftermath of an **ENS** cold or flu, where the **ENS** viral infection has created inflammation that has damaged and dehydrated the mucosal lining of the **Lower Esophageal Sphincter**. Scientists have also explored this same hypothesis as it relates to **GERD** (commonly called heartburn) and have designated it as a significant risk factor in coughs and other pulmonary diseases.[132] My approach, however, does not utilize conventional medicine such as Proton Pump inhibitors but, instead, focuses on restoring the mucosal lining.

With this in mind, I use herbal medicine such as Slippery Elm and Marshmallow Root to address the problem as these natural ingredients help to restore the mucosal lining while also reducing inflammation. Typically, taking a Slippery Elm or Marshmallow Root tea of 1000 mg or four cups several times a day can significantly reduce a cough caused by this problem. Several over-the-counter Slippery Elm cough drops are commercially available and might be helpful as well. However, I find the teas or capsules to be more potent in their effect. Acupuncture in the **ENS** zone can also be useful in helping these kinds of coughs as Acupuncture stimulates blood flow and activates the **Immune Response** to reduce inflammation.[133,134,135,136]

POSTNASAL DRIP COUGH

Postnasal drip or mucousy cough is another common cough that comes after the virus is quelled. These kinds of coughs are a typical symptom of what I call the second phase of the common cold or flu. The symptoms that come with it are much different than the sore throat, fever, and stiff neck found with the first stage of an **ENS** cold or flu. Instead, this phase is dominated by a productive(meaning a cough where you cough up phlegm), hacking cough and postnasal drip.

The prevailing theory is that this phase of a cold or flu indicates that postnasal drip (which is seen as the cause of the cough) is caused by a local **Immune Response** of the mucosal lining of the sinuses. The idea is that because the mucosal lining is inflamed, the **Immune Response** generates mucus to try to combat the infection. However, new evidence points to the problem being related to the bottom-up **Gut-Brain Axis** stress and inflammation, generating mucus that migrates up to the throat and sinuses.

The explanation of how all this mucus accumulates in the gut, at the **Lower Esophageal Sphincter**, is complex. The first thing we need to understand is this problem, in part, is due to a dysfunction of the **Mucosal Immune System**. The **Mucosal Immune System** is the part of the **Immune System** that supports mucus lining throughout our body. The mucosal lining helps to trap pathogens such as viruses, but more importantly, during the second phase of a cold, it helps cleanse the body of all the dead cells from the aftermath of the viral clone wars.

This need for detoxification is particularly relevant to an **ENS** cold or flu, as the **ENS** is embedded in and around the digestive organs and must eventually absorb and break down this debris with the help of the **Immune System**. This detoxification is the defining problem of the second phase of a cold or flu. The detoxification process indicative to the second phase of a cold or flu is also controlled, in part, by the **Immune Response**. However, in the second phase, we must shift our herbal strategy to helping to stimulate the **Immune Response** differently.

In *Chapter 3, Meeting the Challenge of the Clone Wars*, we discussed Th1 versus Th2 immune dominance. We learned that Th1 dominance meant more focus on **Humoral** and **Cell-Mediated Immune dominance**, which is essential for eliminating the virus from our bodies. However, in the second phase, we must shift our attention to Th2 dominance. Th2 means more stimulation of the **Innate Immune Response** and, in particular, **Macrophages**. During the viral stage, **Macrophages** played a different role, engulfing some of the viruses and displaying fragments of the virus on their surfaces to serve as beacons to the **Acquired Immune System**. However, at this stage of the healing process, **Macrophages** play a different role as they engulf pathogens, dead cells, and other cellular waste products. We can think of **Macrophages** as our body's garbage collector, the Janitor Army referenced in *Chapter 3, Meeting the Challenge of the Clone Wars*, and certainly, after a clone war, there are plenty of dead cells and debris to clean up.

Recent studies reveal that **Bile Salts**, a very acidic product of the liver, assist the body in switching to Th2 dominance, which in turn activates the Macrophage garbage collector function. **Bile Salts** are produced in the liver and have been found to perform many vital functions within the **ENS**, including maintaining **Innate** and **Adaptive Immune cells** to regulate **Mucosal Immune** function. Particularly relevant to a postnasal drip cough, **Mucosal Immune** function helps to restore a healthy mucosal environment helping the **ENS** to detoxify the cellular debris from the body's battle from the cold or flu. Detoxification alone can help speed the healing of coughs. Moreover, **Bile Salts** are now understood to be key regulators of microbial colonization in the **Gut Microbiome** due to their ability to stop unhealthy bacteria from growing while promoting the growth of healthy bacteria.

Clearly, **Bile Salts** provide a key way that we are able to fully recover from the second phase of a cold or flu. However, this potent detoxification system is often not functioning well during a cold. There are many factors that contribute to this, but one overarching factor is **Low Vagal Tone** as well as the generalized fatigue that most people experience after fighting off a cold or flu virus.

As **Low Vagal Tone** interferes with the production of **Bile Salts**, the detoxification process is compromised. Add to this, the bottom-up Stress Response, which is also caused by **Low Vagal Tone**. Bottom-up stress means that the **Parasympathetic Nervous System** is partially disabled, leading to an exaggerated pro-inflammatory response. An exaggerated pro-inflammatory response and an inability to rest and digest, places an additional burden on the **Mucosal Immune Response**, adding to the detoxification job of the mucosal lining and **Macrophages**. Seen in this light, coughing seems to be a means that the body bypasses **Low Vagal Tone** by detoxifying excess mucus by coughing it up.

Eventually, most healthy individuals can slowly cough up or absorb the debris of the excess mucus and finally find that their cold or flu is completely healed. This detoxification process can be accelerated by taking herbal products that stimulate **Bile Acids**. Bitter herbs activate the bitter taste receptors, which, in turn, stimulate bile and bile acid production. Bitter taste receptors are located at the back of the tongue and throughout the body and, when activated by herbs with a bitter taste, help stimulate the flow of **Bile Acids**.[137,138,139] Bitter herbs have a long history in Europe and China as an aid to digestion and detoxification. Recently, scientific studies have revealed that they can activate **Bile Salts** and help to reverse the exaggerated pro-inflammatory environment by activating **Vagal Tone**.

Not everyone needs to stimulate **Bile Salts** as part of their recovery from a cold or flu. There is a subset of patients that rarely experience postnasal drip or coughing from too much phlegm. Those people can usually stop after taking their medicinal mushrooms as the second phase of their colds are either nonexistent or so mild that no herbal intervention is required. Below is a questionnaire to help you determine if taking herbs to stimulate **Bile Acids** is appropriate for you.

Health Check

SHOULD I TAKE HERBS TO STIMULATE BILE ACID?

Cough Symptoms (check all that apply):

- ❏ I usually have postnasal drip or a productive cough when I catch a cold or flu.
- ❏ I have Gut Microbiome problems, such as gas, bloating, intermittent diarrhea, loose stool, and/or constipation.
- ❏ I have high cholesterol (emulsifying and ridding the body of cholesterol is one of the functions of **Bile Salts**).
- ❏ I typically feel tired after having oily or greasy food.
- ❏ I tend to suffer from hangovers if I drink.
- ❏ I have a chronic cough where I cough up mucus.
- ❏ I have to avoid certain foods to feel ok.
- ❏ I need more than nine hours of sleep a day.
- ❏ I catch colds easily.
- ❏ It usually takes me three weeks or longer to recover from a cold or flu.

If you have checked two or more items on this list, then you should consider taking herbal bitters, which stimulate Bile Acid production.

HOW TO SUPPORT BILE ACID PRODUCTION

Supporting Bile Acid production is relatively easy using readily available commercial products, usually labeled as Bitters or Swedish Bitters. Bitters are composed of herbs that have a bitter taste. It is their bitter taste that activates the liver to produce Bile and **Bile Salts**. When you start taking one of these products, it's essential to take them in liquid form as the bitter taste is what activates its medicinal benefits. When you start taking these herbs, start with a small dosage, and gradually increase it. I recommend starting with three drops directly in the mouth or in water to see what happens. Within the first day or two, you can usually, through experimentation, find a beneficial dosage. The usual dosage is 5 to 10 drops before eating. If you experience some heartburn, wait for a couple of hours and try taking less. This side effect is unusual, but it's better to start slowly with new herbal medicine and gradually, as you become familiar with its effects, increase it to an optimal dose.

You should feel at least a little more energy and less mucus within minutes of taking this remarkable tonic. With a mucus cough, you can repeat this several times a day.

SUPPORTING THE DETOXIFICATION PROCESS

Detoxification begins almost immediately when you take herbal bitters. In addition to herbal bitters, other simple home therapies support this process. Here are four things other health-related practices you can do:

1. **DRINK PLENTY OF WATER** – up to 8 glasses a day. This helps the body's normal detoxification process happen. Without having enough water, the body cannot properly detoxify.
2. **EAT YOUR VEGGIES** – Antioxidants are abundant in plants and these potent detoxification chemicals help speed the detoxification process.
3. **TAKE HOT BATHS OR SHOWERS** – Soaking in a hot bath or taking a hot shower help the body release toxins through the skin.
4. **AVOID FATTY OR GREASY FOODS** – these place additional burden on Bile Acid production. This is not the time to indulge in eating fried chicken, french fries, or potato chips.

These simple herbal and dietary practices can speed your healing and help you recover from most coughs. If herbal bitters help you with your cough, you can consider incorporating it into your daily supplements, as it will help you stay healthy.

CHAPTER 6
Restore Vagal Tone: Help to Heal Your Bronchitis and Pneumonia

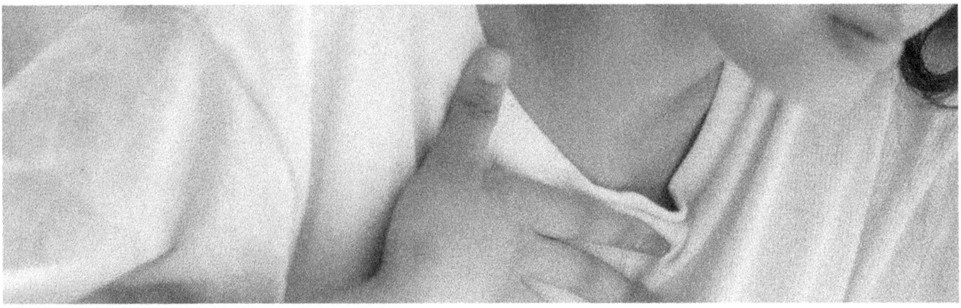

Bronchitis and pneumonia are inflammatory lung disorders that can, especially in the case of pneumonia, develop into serious, even life-threatening illnesses. Bronchitis and pneumonia are often confused as their symptoms are quite similar. Both can result in a productive cough with yellow phlegm, shortness of breath, and fatigue. Bronchitis, however, develops when the bronchial tubes become swollen and inflamed. Pneumonia affects a different part of the lungs, called the alveoli, which become infected and filled with fluid and pus. Below, we'll discuss these illnesses individually, along with what herbs and holistic practices can be used to help them.

Before I discuss these diseases and their differences, I should review **GERD** aspiration as it helps to show the connection of the **Gut-Brain Axis** to these diseases.

GERD AND COUGH

Researchers and doctors have found a strong connection between bronchitis, pneumonia and **GERD**.[140] This connection was investigated when doctors found that patients with **GERD** symptoms had increased risk of developing pulmonary diseases. Interestingly, researchers found this included patients with **GERD** who had no symptoms of heartburn.[141,142] This is what many clinicians are now calling **Silent Reflux**. This relation is another example of how the gastro-intestinal system is implicated in diseases associated with colds and flus, and some of the mechanisms behind an **ENS** viral cold or flu.

BRONCHITIS

Bronchitis literally means inflammation of the bronchial tubes, and the illness is divided into two categories: acute and chronic. Five percent of Americans develop a case of acute bronchitis each year. The primary symptoms of both acute and chronic bronchitis is a cough that is usually productive where yellow phlegm is coughed up. The symptoms of acute bronchitis are:

- A persistent, productive cough.
- Fever.
- Sore throat.
- Wheezing and difficulty breathing.
- A tight chest.
- Body aches.

The symptoms of chronic bronchitis are similar but do not include fever. Also, often chronic bronchitis symptoms don't completely resolve. The symptoms of chronic bronchitis can include:

- A persistent, productive cough that lasts for three weeks or longer.
- Wheezing and difficulty breathing.
- A tight chest.

Acute bronchitis is often associated with the onset of a cold or flu and, because fever and sore throat are among its symptoms, patients should follow the medicinal mushroom herbal protocol found in the *Chapter 3, Meeting the Challenge of the Clone Wars.* Once the fever and sore throat are gone, patients should switch to the bitter herb protocols found in the *Chapter 5, Eliminating Your Cough by Clearing Out Clutter.*

With regard to chronic bronchitis (and even some cases of pneumonia), researchers are now exploring the idea that **Low Vagal Tone** is at least a component of these diseases. After all, **Low Vagal Tone** results in an exaggerated pro-inflammatory response, and increasing **Bile Salts** (which help to restore **Vagal Tone**) increases **Mucosal Immunity**. Boosting **Mucosal Immunity** is particularly helpful as it allows the **Immune Response** to detoxify the debris from the viral cloning wars and, as the mucus lessens, helps to restore **Vagal Tone** and function further.

Coptis, a Chinese herb typically used in TCM clinics all over the world to treat bronchitis, has been identified as a bitter herb that stimulates bile production. I have found this herb to be useful in my clinic for cases for bronchitis with many patients reporting progressive relief of their symptoms. Other bitter herbs such as gentian, dandelion, and globe artichoke should also work as well.

Bitter herbs can be used for a productive cough and should be taken in liquid form, 4 to 8 drops per dose, 4 to 6 times daily. This is the same protocol that I recommend for postnasal drip coughs, which can be referenced in *Chapter 5, Eliminating Your Cough by Clearing Out Clutter.*

PNEUMONIA

Pneumonia is a common illness that affects 450 million people annually worldwide. Pneumonia tends to affect children under five and adults over 70 but can affect patients of any age. It has the potential to be a life-threatening disease, especially in developing countries, and is considered to be one of the leading causes of death in America. Like bronchitis, most pneumonia starts from a viral infection but pneumonia can often develop into a bacterial infection. It is common to catch pneumonia in a hospital setting, and is considered to be the second most common disease acquired at a hospital.

Symptoms of acute pneumonia, mirror those of bronchitis:

- Productive cough with yellow or green mucus.
- Fever.
- Shortness of breath.
- A tight chest.
- Fatigue.

Pneumonia can include symptoms not usually associated with bronchitis:

- Loss of appetite.
- Nausea or vomiting.
- Stabbing chest pain.
- Diarrhea, which is also associated with other acute illnesses like food poisoning or a norovirus intestinal flu.
- A temperature higher than 101 degrees.
- Confusion, spaciness, lack of focus is also found in more advanced cases.

Most cases of pneumonia can respond favorably to the same herbal protocols used for acute or chronic bronchitis. As referenced above, researchers are finding that **Low Vagal Tone** is associated with cases of pneumonia. Because pneumonia can quickly develop into bacterial pneumonia, utilizing a strategy to stimulate **Vagal Tone** can be used to help deter the development of a bacterial pneumonia infection. The primary means that I use to boost **Vagal Tone** is herbal bitters, as bitter herbs help to increase your body's production of **Bile Salts**. **Bile Salts** not only help to improve **Vagal Tone** but also stimulate the Mucosal **Immune System**. Particularly relevant to pneumonia is the bacteriostatic properties that **Bile Salts** offer, which could help lessen the chances of developing bacterial pneumonia while providing a beneficial effect on the **Gut Microbiome**.

While medicinal herbs can be utilized to treat mild to moderate cases of pneumonia, more severe cases where shortness of breath, stabbing chest pains, or high temperatures occur should be referred immediately to a medical doctor or possibly urgent care or the emergency room for hospitalization. Pneumonia with significant shortness of breath or high fever is considered to be a life-threatening disease and prompt medical help is therefore, more appropriate for the treatment of these patients.

In the next section, I have provided a discussion and guidance for herbal treatment for some common symptoms that are found in both bronchitis and pneumonia.

COUGH

For many people with bronchitis or pneumonia, the most bothersome symptom is a chronic phlegmy cough. The herbal protocols explained in *Chapter 5, Eliminating Your Cough by Clearing Out Clutter* can often help a great deal with cough associated with bronchitis and pneumonia. After all, supporting the **Mucosal Immune Response**, activating **Vagal Tone** and the **Parasympathetic Nervous System**, reducing inflammation, supporting the **Gut Microbiome**, and accelerating the detoxification process can help these problems as well. I have many patients with bronchitis who, after 3 or 4 days of taking bitter herbs, indicate that most of their symptoms are gone.

On the other hand, if your symptoms worsen, even when taking herbal medicine, seek medical care. As much as I prefer to avoid referring patients to physicians to get a prescription for antibiotics, antibiotics can be life-saving medicines and should be used in extreme cases. For the vast majority of patients who suffer from bronchitis or mild to moderate pneumonia, these natural protocols can speed the healing process.

GERD AND BRONCHITIS AND PNEUMONIA

Researchers and doctors have found a strong connection between bronchitis, pneumonia and **GERD**.[143] This connection was investigated when doctors found that patients with **GERD** symptoms had increased risk of developing pulmonary diseases. Interestingly, researchers found this included patients with **GERD** with no symptoms of heartburn.[144,145] This is what many clinicians are now calling **Silent Reflux**. This relation is another example of how the gastro-intestinal system is implicated in diseases associated with colds and flus, and some of the mechanisms behind an **ENS** viral cold or flu.

While the connection of **GERD** or **Silent Reflux** to bronchitis and pneumonia is recognized in the medical community as a problem, the use of Proton Pump Inhibitors, which is the usual medicine to address **GERD**, has been found to be ineffective in helping patients with respiratory issues.[146] Instead, if bronchitis or pneumonia is accompanied by **GERD** or **Silent Reflux** symptoms, you should treat these symptoms along with your bronchitis or pneumonia with herbal medicine. If you have **GERD** or **Silent Reflux** symptoms, consider taking Slippery Elm or Marshmallow Root along with bitter herbs. But if you have a fever, you should postpone taking these herbs and instead take medicinal mushrooms until the fever subsides. Once the fever is gone, take 3 to 4 pills of Slippery Elm or Marshmallow Root then, 30 minutes later, follow with 15 drops of a liquid bitter herb mixture. Repeat this up to five times a day.

TIGHT OR PAINFUL CHEST

Some, but not all, patients with bronchitis or pneumonia report a tight or painful chest with some difficulty breathing or shortness of breath. Mild versions of this problem are sometimes due to the displacement of certain intercostal cartilage of the rib cage. Most of the many patients I have seen with this problem report that the issue started as a result of their coughing fits. This condition is similar to another condition called costochondritis. A 2017 study documents the use of cupping to help resolve this condition.

If you feel you have intercostal displacement, you should seek out an acupuncturist who is skilled at cupping and who is capable of palpating and identifying the appropriate area to cup. Usually, one treatment is sufficient to alleviate the chest tightness and sometimes can help restore normal, relaxed breathing. This treatment is for mild symptoms and should not be considered for extreme tension or pain.

SHORTNESS OF BREATH

Shortness of breath is a common symptom that is uncomfortable for a patient and can interfere with the healing process. If a patient's shortness of breath is not severe and is accompanied by chest tightness or pain, I would recommend cupping before you try any additional treatment. As I said before, an acupuncturist must be skilled at cupping and have very good palpation skills. Again, this should only require one or two treatments to get a full resolution of this problem. Manual Osteopathy can sometimes help with mechanical problems involving the rib cage that affect a patient's breathing.

For problems not related to the pinching of spinal nerves within the rib cage, I look at poor lung function due to the build-up of mucus and fluid within the lung. This build up of mucus is often related to poor **Vagal Tone**, which dampens the **Mucosal Immune Response**. Taking herbal bitters may help this problem as **Vagal Tone** not only applies to the **ENS** zone but also the entire **Vagal Nerve** pathway which includes the lungs.

For pneumonia patients who have significant shortness of breath, these herbal recommendations are not appropriate. Severe shortness of breath can be life-threatening. These patients should seek medical care from their doctors or the emergency room at their hospital.

DIARRHEA

Some patients with pneumonia develop diarrhea. These patients should follow the protocols given above but also take probiotics to help restore the bacterial balance of the **Gut Microbiome**. Probiotics tend to be very safe medicines and can provide substantial relief for this problem. In a recent study, administering probiotics to patients with ventilator-associated pneumonia decreased the overall infection in these critically ill patients.[147] Patients with gastrointestinal disease may be more likely to get pneumonia, so taking probiotics should be considered an essential preventative care measure for them. They should take this supplement daily. Also, as **Bile Salts** have been reported to regulate the **Gut Microbiome** bacteria, herbal bitters should be included in patients with this symptom.

For most patients with mild or moderate symptoms, these herbal protocols can provide natural relief of their symptoms and help speed their recovery. I have also found that if patients can stay healthy instead of being plagued by a constant cough or other debilitating symptoms, they are more likely to exercise and make better food choices, thus improving their quality of life all around.

Health Check

WILL SLIPPERY ELM HELP ME?

If you have one of the following symptoms, Slippery Elm may help:

- ❑ A low grade fever
- ❑ Trouble swallowing
- ❑ A lump in your throat
- ❑ A bit of tension in your chest
- ❑ A dry cough that has no fever, or significant sore throat accompanying it

Slippery Elm and/or Marshmallow Root both help to sooth a mild sore throat and lessen a dry cough. Both these herbs help the body to rebuild the mucosal lining of the Lower Esophageal Sphincter and the lining of the esophagus and throat. These herbs are among the mildest herbs available.

WHAT TO DO:

Slippery Elm and Marshmallow Root are available in lozenges, tablets and powders that can make tea. Dosing with capsules, I recommend taking three capsules four to six times a day. The effect of taking these herbs should be apparent within a few minutes of taking them. Take as needed whenever symptoms return.

SIDE EFFECTS:

The mucilaginous phytochemical within these herbs helps the body rebuild the mucosal lining in your body. Because of this property, you should wait at least thirty minutes to an hour after taking one of these supplements before taking any other medicine.

CHAPTER 7

Let the Acetylcholine Flow: How to Open Up Blood and Nerve Flow to Heal a Sinus Infection

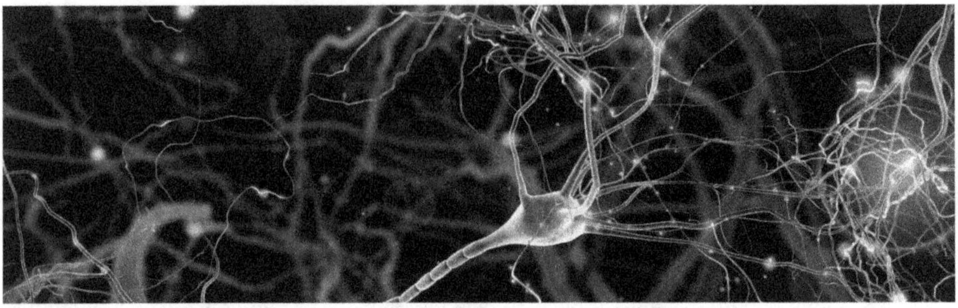

Sinus infections are common in the U.S. In fact, it is reported that 24 to 31 million cases occur in the United States annually.[148] A sinus infection is indicated by the inflammation and swelling of the nasal cavities. Scientists have determined that a particular strain of virus called **Rhinosinusitis** is associated with sinus infections. A sinus infection usually appears during the later stage of a cold, not a flu, and occurs after the sore throat and fever. A cold with a sinus infection may require different treatments from an **ENS** cold. This later stage might have little to do with the original viral infection but instead, be related to a secondary infection, or be related to the stress associated with a cold. To determine the correct course of action, we should look at three types of sinus infections: acute, stress related, and chronic. We will explore the differences between these infections as well as natural treatments for each type in this chapter.

ACUTE SINUS INFECTIONS

An acute sinus infection occasionally occurs together with a severe cold or flu. Patients with acute sinus infections are always very sick and quite miserable, experiencing chills, fever, coughing attacks and very irritated and incessantly runny sinuses. This is a sinus infection related to a virulent strain of a virus and requires frequent dosing of medicinal mushrooms as explained in the instructions found at the end of *Chapter 3, Meeting the Challenge of the Clone Wars.* Also, staying warm and isolating from other people is important in order to recover from this phase of a cold and keep others safe from infection.

STRESS-RELATED SINUS INFECTIONS

This middle stage of a Sinus Infection occurs after much of the viral infection is quelled. The combined problem of continued **ENS** inflammation and a still active **Immune System** (as **T-reg cells** have not yet reversed the **Cell-Mediated Immune Response**[149]), amplifies **Low Vagal Tone**, resulting in poor conduction in the Vagus Nerve.

This temporary Immune-Stress-Neurological dysfunction stimulated by an **ENS** viral infection creates an **Acetylcholine** shunt that starves muscles along the **Vagal Nerve** pathway causing these muscles to temporarily stiffen. As we learned in the *Chapter 2, Second Brain* and *Chapter 4, The Body's Secret Regulator*, this causes the back of the neck to become stiff, as well as slightly compressing the trigeminal cranial nerve that exits at the junction of the neck and head.

This cranial nerve frequently becomes pinched as a result of low tone of the **Trigeminal Nerve** causing the muscles surrounding the sinuses to suffer not only from poor nerve conduction but also poor blood circulation. All this shunting of **Acetylcholine** and the tension directly over the sinus area of the face, leads to sinus congestion, pressure and poor blood flow. The latter problem creates an environment conducive for viral evasion. More information on the **Trigeminal Nerve** can be found in *Chapter 2, Second Brain.*

VIRUS MIGRATION

While I believe the vast majority of colds and flus start in the **ENS** zone, I do think that viruses can migrate to the lungs and sinuses. As the **B-cells**, **T-cells** and **NK cells** slowly eliminate the virus from our system, the sinuses and lungs can remain infected simply because the nerve flow and muscle tension contribute to poor blood flow in these areas. This restricts the flow of **white blood cells** to these areas and creates a log jam in the process hindering the complete elimination from the body of the virus. Add to this the fact that **Vagal Tone**, at the middle stage of a cold, is often still low, and **T-reg cells** have yet to turn down the **Immune Response**, the resulting in a sinus infection that can continue for days or weeks even after most of the virus has been eliminated.

EXCESS MUCOUS

Along with **Low Vagal Tone**, compressed cranial nerves and poor blood flow, the hallmark of a sinus infection is the copious amounts of mucous suffered by the infected. Many people mistakenly believe that the sinuses, under siege from a pathogen such as a virus, generate copious amounts of mucus as part of the **Immune Response**. However, given the poor blood and nerve flow to the sinuses, a substantial local **Immune Response** is unlikely.

The mucus actually comes from the debris created during the cloning war between the **Immune System** and the viral replicas taking place within the **ENS**. As I said in the *Chapter 3, Meeting the Challenge of the Clone Wars,* the immune cells must literally kill off millions of our own cells in order to eliminate the virus that has hijacked them, and much of this debris is removed within the mucus that is formed in this killing process.

Much of this **Immune System** battle happens at ground zero, in and around the **Lower Esophageal Sphincter**. The **ENS** remains inflamed for days partly due to the extensive cleanup operation underway to get rid of all the dead cells. It should not be surprising that this process generates a lot of mucous, aided by a temporarily compromised **Lower Esophageal Sphincter**, allowing much of this mucous to migrate up the esophagus to the throat and sinuses. This mucus is usually experienced by patients as post-nasal drip and a runny, stuffy nose.

A final piece of the puzzle is being revealed in recent research. It seems that **ENS** function and proper regulation of the **Immune Response** is, in part, controlled by **Bile Acids**,[150,151] which are generated by the liver and stored in the gallbladder. I have reviewed the role of **Bile Acids** and the Immune function in more depth in the *Chapter 5, Eliminating Your Cough by Clearing Out Clutter.* The bottom line is that the body needs increased **Bile Acids** during this time to regulate the **Immune Response**, and bitter herbs, which activate **Bile Acids** via the bitter taste receptors, are therefore a powerful natural method to treat sinus infections.

WHAT TO DO

1. **ADDRESS LOW VAGAL TONE** – Acupuncture Osteopathic manual therapy such as Visceral Massage, or topical Shinus Molle can all help to restore Vagal Tone and help reduce the body's Stress Response and relax tense neck muscles.

2. **HELP REDUCE THE INFLAMMATION OF THE LOWER ESOPHAGEAL SPHINCTER** – Take Slippery Elm or Marshmallow Root in capsules or tea. This only works when the fever and sore throat have abated.
3. **HAVE A HEALTHCARE PROFESSIONAL FURTHER LOOSEN THE NECK AND CRANIAL BONE RESTRICTIONS** that are reducing nerve conduction into the sinuses. The usual healthcare professionals that work on this problem include specially-trained Acupuncturists, Osteopaths knowledgeable in manual medicine, a trusted upper-cervical Chiropractor, or a specially-trained Physical Therapist. From my experience, one or two sessions should be sufficient to help open the sinuses and help restore blood flow to and proper functioning of the sinuses.
4. **TAKE BITTER HERBS** to help detoxify and flush the dead cell debris from the body. In TCM, this go-to formulation is called Bi Yan Wan, which includes herbs such as magnolia bud, cocklebur and coptis. Coptis is the most important herb in this formulation as it is bitter and has both antibiotic and antifungal properties. There is something unique about the TCM formulation that seems to be especially effective against this middle stage of sinus infections. Swedish Bitters can also be helpful.
5. **DRINK PLENTY OF WATER** – Hydration is also key to help speed the detoxification process.

CHRONIC AND RECURRENT SINUS INFECTIONS

Chronic recurrent sinus infections are sinus infections that either last much longer than a normal cold or are infections that occur four or more times per cold season. Often a thick yellow discharge, sinus congestion, and pain and swelling are key symptoms, and at times some will report sinus headaches. The cause of these sinus infections is controversial as many bacteria and fungus are present when cultured. However, treating with antibiotics or antifungal medicines have been found to be ineffective. The prestigious *Cochrane Review* did a meta-study review of quality studies regarding antibiotic therapy and concluded that there is "very little evidence that systemic antibiotics are effective in patients with chronic **Rhinosinusitis**."[152]

My many years of experience using acupuncture and herbs, along with the experience of my Osteopathic colleagues, has resulted in promising results. There are several positive studies of Acupuncture for allergic rhinitis[153] and one small study showing benefits of Osteopathic manual medicine.[154] More studies are needed, but the approach listed above for stress-related Sinusitis is often helpful in these cases. Below I will list exactly what I recommend to help get rid of this chronic condition.

WHAT TO DO

1. **ADDRESS LOW VAGAL TONE** with Acupuncture and Osteopathic manual manipulations.
2. **HELP REDUCE THE INFLAMMATION OF THE LOWER ESOPHAGEAL SPHINCTER** using Slippery Elm or Marshmallow Root capsules or tea.
3. **TAKE BI YAN WAN** or other bitter herbs several times a day.
4. **HAVE A HEALTHCARE PROFESSIONAL FURTHER LOOSEN THE NECK AND CRANIAL BONE RESTRICTIONS** that are reducing nerve conduction into the sinuses. The usual healthcare professionals that work on this problem include specially-trained Acupuncturists, Osteopaths knowledgeable in manual medicine, a trusted upper-cervical Chiropractor, or a specially-trained Physical Therapist. From my experience, one or two sessions should be sufficient to help open the sinuses and help restore blood flow and proper functioning to the sinuses.
5. **ADDRESS POSSIBLE TMJ PROBLEMS** using cupping or Osteopathic manipulation. The Trigeminal Nerve passes through the TMJ area which can compromise the nerve conduction of this cranial nerve and lead to the tightening of muscle overlying the sinuses.
6. **TRY SALINE SINUS IRRIGATION** through a neti pot or over-the-counter saline irrigation bottle several times a day.
7. **HAVE YOUR GUT MICROBIOME AND STOMACH EVALUATED** as these problems can interfere with the **Immune System**'s ability to fight off an infection as well as create chronic **Low Vagal Tone**. You can use the questionnaire provided in *Chapter 4, The Body's Secret Regulator* as a preliminary evaluation. There are certain healthcare professionals that specialize in this area who can assist you in healing this problem.

8. **TAKE HERBAL BITTERS** to activate the **Immune Response**. An example of an herbal formulation with bitter properties is **Bi Yan Wan**.
9. **DRINK PLENTY OF WATER**.

Other measures listed above are for those who want to address this problem in a more complete way. Patients who find that even these steps only partially help their problem should be evaluated for other sinus-related problems such as sinus polyps or a deviated septum. These problems can often improve using holistic steps listed above but may, ultimately, require surgery.

For allergic rhinitis, all the above steps except for **Bi Yan Wan** may be helpful. Instead of **Bi Yan Wan**, the go-to herbal remedy for an allergy is called **Pe Men Kan Wan**, which is specific for frequent sneezing and a constant runny nose.

CHAPTER 8
Taking Control: What You Can Do For The Novel Coronavirus, COVID-19

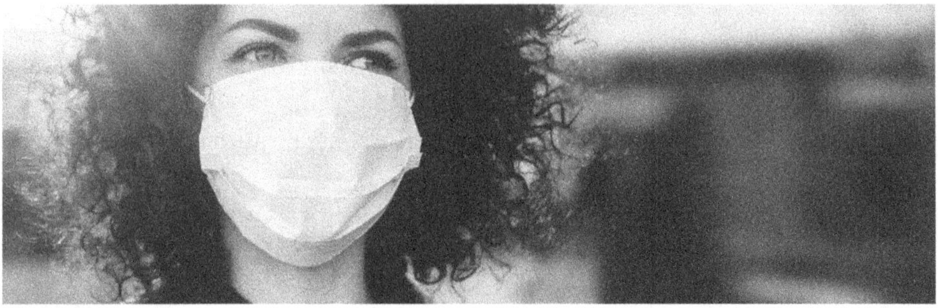

Every decade or so, we encounter a new super virus that spreads far more rapidly and is far more lethal than the flu. In 2004, the SARS-CoV virus emerged as a pandemic virus that was a strain of the Coronavirus. This outbreak, however, was contained early and did not create the global disruption of the current COVID-19 virus, although in the end it had a higher fatality rate (11%) with 8,096 total confirmed cases. At the writing of this book, the Coronavirus COVID-19 has reached pandemic proportions and, as of March 2020, has grown to over 1,380,000 confirmed cases and thousands of deaths. It is creating chaos and havoc in the social fabric, healthcare and finances of the world. These super virus symptoms can be mild but, for the elderly or immunocompromised, the symptoms can be quite severe and even deadly. Here are some of the striking differences between the common flu virus and these more lethal strains:

SYMPTOMS

Symptoms of COVID-19 are more or less typical of any flu. This list provides the most common symptoms to the least common symptoms:

- Fever.
- Dry Cough.
- Fatigue.
- Coughing up thick phlegm.
- Shortness of breath.
- Muscle or joint pain.

- Sore throat.
- Headache.
- Chills.
- Nausea or Vomiting.
- Nasal Congestion.
- Diarrhea.
- Temporary loss of smell and/or taste.

TRANSMISSION

One of the defining characteristics of a pandemic is that it is much more easily spread than the typical flu or cold. In the case of COVID-19, scientists now believe each infected patient will infect an average of 2 to 2.5 additional people. A patient infected with the flu only spreads the virus to an average of 1.3 other people.

WHAT IS THE BEST PREVENTATIVE MEASURE?

As this virus is 2 to 2.5 times as contagious as a typical cold or flu virus, isolation of anyone infected with COVID-19 is critically important. Social distancing is deemed essential by the CDC to prevent the spread of this and other viral infections. Social distancing means maintaining a distance of at least 6 feet between yourself and others. Also, it means avoiding crowds or enclosed spaces with other people, such as an elevator or an airplane.

A face mask should be worn by anyone who has to travel outside of their home. Besides a face mask, everyone should consider wearing some kind of protective eyewear, whether they are sunglasses or normal glasses, as viruses can be transmitted through any part of the body that has a mucus membrane, including the eyes. Healthcare workers, for instance, are required to wear protective eyewear.

Other hygiene practices highly relevant to preventing catching this virulent virus are reviewed in *Chapter 1, Hijacked.*

HOW SEVERE ARE COVID-19 SYMPTOMS AND WHEN SHOULD I SEEK CARE?

Public health officials categorize COVID-19 symptoms as mild, severe, and critical. Let us look at the data that is currently available.

Mild Cases

Early studies from China show that 81% of reported cases were mild.[155] These cases had milder symptoms with no or mild pneumonia. The typical recovery time is reported as averaging two weeks.

Severe Cases

Severe cases had much more severe symptoms such as significant shortness of breath, low oxygen levels and/or more significant levels of fluid (including pus, blood and/or protein) in the lungs. Fourteen percent of patients were reported as having severe COVID-19 symptoms.[156]

Critical Cases

These patients have life-threatening symptoms such as septic shock, respiratory failure and/or organ failure. Five percent of patients were listed as being critical.[157]

CURRENT CONVENTIONAL TREATMENT

The medical world is desperately seeking a viable treatment of this new virus. It seems unlikely that any new drug or vaccination will emerge soon. While there are a few antiviral medications that can be used to fight this flu, they are rarely used. One concern is that viruses are highly adaptive and as they go through rapid replication, can easily mutate to a slightly different form.[158] This creates problems for those developing antiviral drugs because as the virus mutates it becomes resistant to the drug. Moreover, no antiviral drug is currently. In addition to this problem of virus evolution, the CDC states that "antiviral treatment works best when started soon after flu illness begins. When antiviral treatment is started within two days of becoming sick with flu symptoms, these drugs can lessen fever and flu symptoms and shorten the time you are sick by about one day."[159] As is typical for a novel virus, no vaccine is available for this strain of the flu.

USING HERBAL MEDICINE TO COMBAT COVID-19

Mild Cases

The data shown above indicates that 81% of the reported cases are categorized as mild. These cases are appropriate for immune stimulation using medicinal mushrooms, as outlined in *Chapter 3, Meeting the Challenge of the Clone Wars*. Topical Schinus Molle in the epigastric region is also recommended. This immune stimulation should be continued until the fever and sore throat are gone. (Note: only 13.9% of COVID-19 patients report having a sore throat). Within two to four days of following this protocol, patients should find a significant improvement of their symptoms. This means that at least mild cases of COVID-19 should respond to immune stimulation in a similar way to a standard seasonal flu.

After the fever and sore throat are gone, patients can switch to taking bitters and probiotics according to directions provided in *Chapter 5, Eliminating Your Cough by Clearing Out Clutter*. This herbal protocol is helpful in order to stimulate **Vagal Tone**, which will help mitigate bottom-up stress. Moreover, it helps reverse the exaggerated pro-inflammatory **Mucosal Immune Response** and helps to restore **Gut Microbiome** bacterial balance. More importantly, bitters can help to stimulate **Bile Salts**, which then provide intrinsic bacteriostatic properties that should help to deter the development or at least progression of pneumonia. All of these beneficial effects are reviewed in more detail in *Chapter 5, Eliminating Your Cough by Clearing Out Clutter* as well as *Chapter 6, Restore Vagal Tone.*

Severe Cases

The same protocols can be applied for those who have severe COVID-19 symptoms, as defined by the World Health Organization. Immune stimulation followed by restoring **Vagal Tone** using bitter herbs can, at least for some, be enough to help through this more severe set of symptoms. I would recommend that patients continue this protocol as long as it is reducing their fever, chills, body aches, and/or sore throat. If there is no improvement after 24 to 48 hours of taking the appropriate herbs, then it is time to abandon what I call Plan A and go to Plan B. Plan B means seeking conventional medical care. Plan B especially applies to those who have shortness of breath or difficulty breathing.

Critical Cases

It is not appropriate or responsible to use immune stimulation with herbs for those with any of the critical symptoms shown above. These patients will need the care of a medical team with access to respirators, oxygen, and other medications and protocols for handling life-threatening emergencies. Often patients who have a critical diagnosis have other severe health conditions which complicate the treatment and require medical professionals who are expert in emergency treatments. If you have critical symptoms, put this book down and go to the hospital.

MORTALITY

COVID-19 currently has a 3.4% mortality rate, and the flu has less than 1%. SARS-CoV, on the other hand, had a mortality rate of 10%.[160] The numbers here are based on current best estimates and will be updated as more data is available.

CAN THIS HERBAL PROTOCOL WORK FOR A PANDEMIC VIRUS?

Immune stimulation, including herbal immune stimulation, is currently an area of interest to the scientific community in addressing superbugs such as COVID-19. In particular, there is much discussion of the **NK cells** as a key Immune cell that helps the body kill infected cells. New studies also show that these superbugs target and attack **NK cells**, so it makes sense to stimulate the production of these cells to help cytotoxic warriors fight off the replication of this virus. The key to success using herbal medicine to boost immunity, in my view, is to maintain a high level of **NK cells** so that the numbers of virally-infected cells continues to decline.

After the initial assault of the COVID-19 virus, it is equally important to stimulate **Vagal Tone** as this stage is particularly crucial in any influenza, including COVID-19, where patients tend to develop pneumonia or a cough. More research is needed in this area to assess this strategy. Still, given my success with using this approach with hundreds of patients with other viral strains of colds and cases of flu, I believe that this provides a safe and effective means to combat this virus and could provide real answers to the devastating problems that COVID-19 is creating.

APPENDIX A
How Chinese Medicine Diagnoses and Treats the Common Cold and Flu

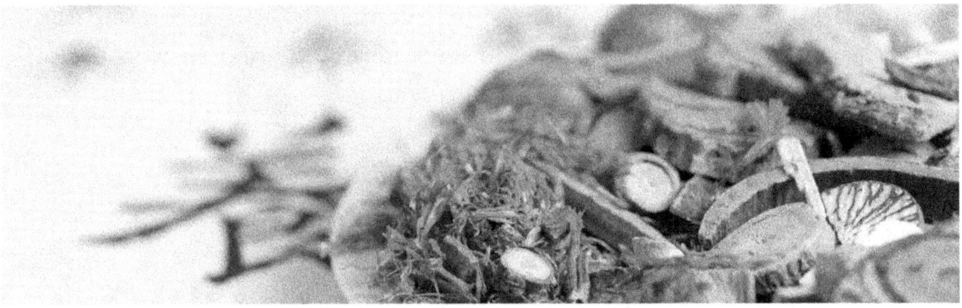

ENVIRONMENTAL CAUSES AND PATTERNS

Traditional Chinese Medicine (**TCM**) physicians routinely treat patients with colds or flus. In fact, Asian physicians have been diagnosing and treating the common cold with herbs and acupuncture since the beginning of **TCM**, more than two thousands years ago. Today, **TCM** is widely used throughout Asia and the West as it has been shown to give patients considerable relief from their colds and flu. Given the history of **TCM**, it may not be surprising that the precepts, diagnoses and treatments were developed long before the modern scientific discovery of cold viruses or secondary bacterial infections. While **TCM** developed without the benefits of these and many other modern discoveries and concepts, it has entered the modern world with surprising and helpful medical treatments for the common cold and flu in Asia, and is now becoming more popular in the West.

Developed through trial and error, this system, early on, appointed committees to collect data on herbal approaches to repeat and confirm the findings. Chinese physicians then collated this information into reference manuals, which provided herbal protocols and diagnostic principles that formulated the protocols and principles of **TCM** diagnosis and treatment. Ultimately, through the course of hundreds of years, **TCM** understanding and practice has been refined and documented in thousands of texts and clinical manuals which show the effectiveness as well as the evolution of this medicine through time. Old **TCM** text books such as the Yellow Emperor's Classic can be found along with their modern counterparts in **TCM** libraries providing herbal compendiums, acupuncture methods and prescriptions, case studies and many other functions of this medical system. These texts provide a continuous record of medical inquiry since it was first taught to Asian **TCM** medical students in the 7th century. This long-standing medical educational system has helped to make **TCM** the most extensively documented and studied medical tradition found in natural medicine.

Its history, including its extensive documentation, makes **TCM** stand out in the world medical arena. Combining that with thousands of modern medical studies, which serve to validate **TCM** methods and treatments, has satisfied even the World Health Organization (WHO) of its efficacy. The WHO has designated **TCM** as an appropriate treatment for colds and flus (among many other medical conditions).[161]

As more scientific scrutiny is directed to **TCM**, additional findings and insights continue to add to the evolution of **TCM**. In fact, many of the common phytochemicals (natural chemicals found within Asian medicinal herbs) have been scientifically studied, and it has been discovered that many herbs can inhibit viruses that cause the common cold and influenza. In addition to this vital effect, many herbs used to treat colds and flus also increase immune response, reduce inflammation, increase blood flow to the infected areas, and help with a myriad of other problems associated with the cold and flu. Studies of phytochemicals such as Quercetin,[162,163] Apegin and Andrographolide, which are found in many herbs used to treat colds and flus demonstrate inhibitory effects against the viruses, and demonstrate that **TCM** has passed through more scientific scrutiny.

Many western physicians now believe that **TCM** stands to fully enter the modern world, where the ancient precepts that **TCM** was founded upon can be combined with scientific research forming the foundation of new, science-based protocols and procedures. I have, with this book, begun the quest to bring the refined lens of science to this medical system. My focus, rather than working with herbs that inhibit viral replication, is to instead place attention on Immune Stimulation and modulation of Vagal Tone and the Gut Microbiome. It can be quite instructive to examine the principles and practice of **TCM** in regards to colds and flus. I can honestly say that I have not discarded this elegant system of diagnosis and treatment, but rather use it as a frame of reference for much of my investigations.

PRINCIPLES OF TCM AND THE COMMON COLD AND FLU

The theory of **TCM** is based on scientific principles of observation, evaluation, treatment, and follow-up. One of the most important steps in this process is taking an account of every aspect of the patient's cold or flu including the onset, cause and symptoms that are reported. Using these principles to diagnose a cold or flu can be quite helpful in choosing the correct herbal and acupuncture prescriptions rather than just picking out herbs from a list "that are good for colds." Included in this scientific process is asking a patient how they caught their cold or flu.

Often patients report that they caught a cold or flu after being chilled or exposed to cold damp weather. Interestingly, for Chinese Medical theory, cold and damp weather are seen as causes of catching a cold. While this has been proven to be incorrect, modern science has determined that viruses become more viable in cold weather.[164] Moreover, the Chinese also included other weather conditions such as excessively dry or hot weather as potential causes. Other considerations include detailing the symptoms and objective signs such as the rate and quality of the pulse.

It's remarkable that a medical system still exists where your experience of "what happened" and which symptoms you have figures into the equation of how you are treated. If, for instance, you say that you "got chilled" and, as a result, have a sore throat, stuffy nose, slight fever, and fatigue, the Chinese physician writes this down as important information, noting all your symptoms and tailoring your herbal formula and acupuncture treatment accordingly. In this appendix, I will provide information on the main **TCM** patterns that form the theoretical framework through which you can find the most helpful treatment to speed the healing of a cold or flu. You will soon find that these patterns form a very logical and helpful manner to find appropriate treatments that are particularly suited to selecting the right herbs to help you and your family.

Below, I describe the Five Environmental Causes (EC) that, according to **TCM**, cause the common cold. These environmental causes are also used as the names of the disease patterns. For example, if a person is exposed to "the cold" (meaning they have been exposed to cold weather), they can develop "a Cold" (the disease) and should be treated accordingly. The same applies to damp or excessively dry weather. Let us explore the Five Environmental Causes of colds and flus.

THE FIVE ENVIRONMENTAL PATTERNS

The five causes which negatively influence the body causing disharmony and disease are:

- Exposure to cold.
- Exposure to wind.
- Heat (inflammation).
- Dampness (excessive mucus and/or swelling).
- Dryness (dehydration and/or damage to the mucosal linings).

Together, these Five Environmental causes form the core of the diagnostic system in **TCM**.

EXPOSURE TO COLD

We all instinctively know that cold weather brings the risk of catching a cold. In cold weather, we bundle up in warm clothing to go outside. Children especially seem vulnerable to "catching a chill" if they are not properly dressed for freezing weather. Most of us have had the experience of being exposed to a cold snap and then ending up with getting a head or chest cold. **TCM** physicians noted the same phenomenon and designated this as a cause of catching a cold. In fact, the **TCM** exposure to cold is most commonly associated with any illness that results in exposure to a cold draft. This means that in **TCM**, being exposed to cold weather or chilling the body by any means, often precipitates the onset of a cold. This could be swimming in cold water or sleeping on a cold floor or bed or being exposed to air-conditioning that is so cold that you feel chilled from it. In **TCM**, we say that "cold" enters the body through the back of the neck, the soles of the feet and the palms of the hands. However, these represent only the most vulnerable areas of the body, which means that exposure to cold can happen to any part of the body at any point.

Many medical authorities believe that the reason people living in cold climates catch colds more frequently is because they are confined indoors and therefore, in closer proximity to infected people. However, little or no research has been done to verify this opinion. Looking at it from a physiological point of view, there are valid reasons that exposure to cold could predispose us to catching a cold. First, the cold and flu viruses are more viable in cold weather. Additionally, cold weather causes a kind of overall stress, tightening muscles and restricting the intake of air. This kind of stress not only restricts muscles and ultimately circulation, but also serves to lower the immune system response to viruses. This closely corresponds to what we say in **TCM**, that the cold invades the Meridians or channels in the body, constricting them and leading to pain and limiting function of the organs, especially the lungs and the nervous system.

The Cold Pattern

Cold is not only an environmental cause of the common cold, but it is also the name given to a certain constellation of symptoms in **TCM** which are caused by exposure to cold weather. Below, I have listed the cold symptoms individually. These symptoms, however, should be viewed as a collective whole. This does not mean that every symptom below must be present in order to diagnose this pattern, but only that there is a lot of overlap in symptom identification in **TCM**, which means we must look at the whole picture before we can identify a pattern. This method of looking at the whole picture is common to all of the environmental patterns.

The symptoms of the Cold Pattern are:

1. Chills along with fever.
2. A thin, watery, clear sinus discharge or post-nasal drip.
3. Some fatigue and general malaise.
4. Joint or body pain (this is due to cold invading the meridians).

To give a more graphic picture of a patient with Cold Pattern symptoms: they cannot seem to get warm and even shiver with cold; have a runny nose; and their body feels sore and uncomfortable. These patients may be treated with herbal treatments and Moxa. Moxa is a herb (Mugwort) that is burned over acupuncture points to warm and bring more circulation to the body.

Influenza outbreaks also occur seasonally in the winter. This is thought to be because people spend more time indoors and thus in more close proximity, promoting increased person-to-person transmission. Additionally, the virus survives longer on surfaces at colder temperatures.[165]

Treatment of Someone Who Has Symptoms From Exposure to Cold

Chills and Body Ache

Modern research shows that Ephedra, Dried Ginger Root, Peony Root, Licorice, and Cinnamon Root are vasodilating, which would help with a cold condition.[166,167]

From a **TCM** perspective, herbal medicines for colds include warming herbs that induce a mild diaphoresis (sweating) tend to be very soothing and typically provide significant symptom relief from this type of cold.

Runny Nose (Clear Discharge)

Xanthium and Magnolia Bud are utilized for any runny nose condition, including allergies, and tend to be quite effective. Some research has documented the effectiveness of these herbs in sinus conditions.[168,169] There are research articles that document a **TCM** herbal formula with several herbs which include Xanthium and Magnolia Bud as the primary herbs.[170,171]

Acupuncture or Acupressure

MOXA ON LI4, ST36 , GB20 AND REN 10

Utilize Moxa sticks to heat the points. These treatments should be administered by qualified TCM practitioners to ensure that the points are heated without burning the patient.

MOXA (OR MOXIBUSTION)

Moxa is a heating method used in TCM to heat acupuncture points to deeply warm the body and/or stimulate blood flow to certain areas of the body. Typically, an herb found throughout the world called Mugwort is used. A small amount of the dried herb is placed on the skin or in a large cigar shaped stick and lit with fire. It is then quickly removed when it starts to burn the skin. The effects can be quite pleasant for someone with cold extremities or who is suffering from the Cold Pattern.

Side effects can include skin burns, especially when Moxa is not removed from the skin quickly enough, and smoke allergy symptoms for those who are sensitive to Moxa smoke.

Treatment Results

Treatment should provide symptom relief in a short period of time. The cold symptoms will often partially resolve and the individual may recover sooner. However, this type of cold, at least in my practice, is not common and so, these treatments are rarely utilized. In Integrative Medicine, people susceptible to cold weather or drafts are evaluated as having endocrine problems, poor circulation and/or poor immunity. These can all be treated holistically and, once improved, can help people prevent catching a cold. Herbal and Moxa treatments can and should be utilized for symptom relief when the patient's symptoms are significant chills or runny nose.

Possible Side Effects of Herbal Treatment

Those utilizing Moxa treatment must be careful to apply this heating technique with care or else there is a risk of burning the skin. Also, if this treatment is utilized for the wrong symptom pattern, there is a risk of increased fever, or a sore throat. Cold Pattern treatments are contraindicated for those with a sore throat or fever. Ephedra is now banned by the FDA as a stimulant as it appears to stimulate norepinephrine (a form of adrenaline), and, when taken excessively, can result in heart palpitations, insomnia, anxiety, and in rare cases death. Some Western allergy over-the-counter (OTC) medicines that remain on the market also stimulate the same norepinephrine and can cause the identical side effects. Other herbs can have minor side effects such as dry mouth or indigestion for those that are allergic to them.

EXPOSURE TO WIND

The Exposure to Wind Pattern is associated with exposure to windy weather. It can also apply to exposure to the air flow from air conditioning or a fan. Wind symptoms are common to colds as well as environmental allergies and, according to **TCM**, perpetuate other conditions in the lungs and upper abdomen.

Windy days, especially when it's cold, can quickly dehydrate and chill our bodies and bring on cold. Wind in **TCM** has a unique constellation of symptoms as shown below.

Wind Pattern

- Sneezing, itchy throat, nose, eyes or ears.
- Transient, migrating pain symptoms moving through the body (pain that tends to migrate from a headache to a stiff neck).
- Rapid onset of symptoms.

In **TCM**, the Wind Pattern is rarely viewed by itself. Instead, it is most often combined with other patterns. For instance, the Cold Pattern or Heat Pattern (described below) combined with the Wind Pattern can create a combined set of symptoms. The combination of Wind and Cold Patterns is called "Wind-Cold" and the combination of Wind and Heat Patterns is called "Wind-Heat." Below is a list of symptoms of these combined Wind-Cold and Wind-Heat patterns.

Wind-Cold Pattern:

- Rapid onset of symptoms.
- Sneezing.
- Feeling chilled (although it's actually a fever).
- Itchy throat.
- Mild headache that migrates from one part of the head to another.
- Body and joint pain that can be sharp and comes and goes.

Wind-Heat is a bit confusing as it has come to represent a cold with more inflammatory symptoms rather than exposure to hot weather or prolonged heat. Combining symptoms of inflammation to the Wind Pattern produces additional symptoms such as a sore throat and fever.

Wind-Heat Pattern

- Rapid onset of symptoms.
- Fever of 99-105°.
- Sore throat.
- Mild headache with migrating pain.
- Red eyes.
- Increased thirst.
- Fatigue.
- Pulse is floating and fast.
- Transient pain and changeable symptoms.

These two categories, Wind-Cold and Wind-Heat, provide a view of the **TCM** models for the first onset of a cold. The Wind-Cold pattern begins with sneezing and feeling chilled. In **TCM** we often suggest that when Wind-Cold symptoms begin, these patients must immediately rest and hope that their immune system rallies so they can fend off the cold. Keeping warm is crucial to recovery.

Wind-Heat is an alternative first stage of a cold which can be more difficult to recover from and more uncomfortable for the patient. Wind Heat includes more serious symptoms such as sore throat and fever. This pattern implies that people are confined to bed and feel quite lethargic and unable to function in any but the most basic activities. The difference in treatment and prognosis for these two patterns in **TCM** is remarkably different and demonstrates the specificity and power of this approach. Below we will give an overview of the treatments for these two types of Wind Patterns.

Treatment of Wind-Cold and Wind-Heat Patterns

WIND-COLD Sneezing, chilled, itchy throat	WIND-HEAT Sore throat, mild headache, fever, fatigue
Gui Zhi Tang, comprised of the following herbs: Cinnamon, White Peony, Fresh Ginger, Jujube, and Honey Fried Licorice.	Honeysuckle Flower, Forsythia, Isatis Root, Andrographis and Echinacea *Herbal formulas including Gan Mao Ling and Yin Qiao San are typical patent herbal medicines available in pill form.* *Gan Mao Ling and Yin Qiao San herbal Wind-Heat formulas are the most common traditional TCM cold formulas for treating colds. Gan Mao Ling is perhaps the most widely used cold remedy in China and Taiwan.*
Large Intestine 4, Gall Bladder 20	Lung 10, Lung 5, Stomach 44

Home Care

WIND-COLD Sneezing, chilled, itchy throat	WIND-HEAT Sore throat, mild headache, fever, fatigue
Keep the patient warm, even using heating pads or Moxa.	Take tea brewed from herbs shown above up to 10 times a day.
Take herbs 3 to 4 times daily.	

Integrative Comments

While I have a great deal of respect for **TCM** and this nuanced approach to treating the beginning stages of the cold, I only rarely utilize these categories or treatments in my clinic anymore. I have included them, however, to present to you the comprehensive system used in **TCM** and the thoughtful systematic treatment that has been used over hundreds of years. Also, this system provided the seminal understanding that allowed me to analyze colds in a different and helpful way that eventually led me to a new understanding. While Wind-Heat appears to be a description of what we now call a typical upper-respiratory infection, my scientific approach to treating colds and flus naturally has led me in a different direction.

HEAT (INFLAMMATION) PATTERN

Heat, or simply hot weather, as an environmental factor is not considered to be a true cause of the common cold. It is, however, a concept in **TCM** associated with inflammation. When it comes to the common cold, it is more useful to think of it simply as a cold with inflammatory symptoms. Inflammation is a very useful element when categorizing a cold or flu, and has several subcategories in the **TCM** system. Above I reviewed the signs and symptoms of Wind-Heat but there are actually several cold types that have heat as one of the cofactors. The most basic heat category in **TCM** is called Lung Heat, which indicates that the lungs are inflamed and presents as a very basic cold pattern.

Lung Heat

Lung Heat symptoms are common at the onset of a cold, especially a child's cold, with usually only four symptoms present:

- A moderate fever 100-103°.
- The tip of the tongue is quite red.
- Excessive thirst.
- Red face or red rash on face.
- No sore throat.

Lung Heat indicates that the lungs are inflamed and the moderate fever shows that the body's innate immune system is engaged while the anti-inflammatory acquired immune system has yet to kick in. (See the Immune System chapter for more information about the acquired immune system). The Lung Heat symptoms are similar to Wind Heat pattern, however, a person is usually not as sick and debilitated with Lung Heat as they are with Wind Heat. Lung Heat is sometimes helpful in treating children under six.

Treatment of Lung Heat Pattern

LUNG HEAT
Gardenia, Coptis, Scutellaria, Rhubarb *These herbs tend to help reduce inflammation related to a cold and can be helpful in this beginning phase of a cold.*
Large Intestine 11, Lung 10, ST 44

Integrative Medicine Comments

The Primary herbal formula to treat Lung Heat symptoms is called Huang Hian Shang Qing Wan. It has Gardenia, Coptis and other herbs that reduce the lung inflammation and bring quick relief to a child or adult with this set of symptoms.

Wind Heat

Wind Heat is a second heat category.

Heat Toxin

Heat Toxin is a specific kind of heat or inflammation that is caused by a toxin. In modern **TCM** theory it is widely believed that this category is associated with viruses and in some cases, secondary bacterial infections.

The symptoms of Heat Toxin are as we might expect from any viral inflammation such as more intense sore throat and malaise. A higher fever is also indicative of Heat Toxin. These symptoms are due to the pathogen infecting the cells in the throat, sinus and upper respiratory tract.

Symptoms include:

- Sore and/or burning throat.
- Redness in the throat and/or tonsils.
- Burning sensation of the lungs.
- High fever.
- Yellow and/or green sinus mucus.

Heat toxin is presumed to be part of any virulent cold including Wind Heat colds so there is a common herbal strategy that may be added to other **TCM** patterns such as Damp Heat or **Tai Yang** colds. Heat Toxin has become more important in **TCM** since the discovery of viruses and secondary bacterial infections and illustrates how **TCM** has evolved over time.

Below I have listed the most common **TCM** and Western herbs that are included in this category.

Treatment of Heat Toxin

HEAT TOXIN
Honeysuckle with Forsythia, Istatis, Ilex Root, Andrographis, Echinacea (alcohol extract)[172]
While not a Chinese herb, many practitioners put this herb in the Heat Toxin category.
Usnea[173]

Shinus Molle

A well-known South American herb that is gaining a lot of attention with herbalists as providing potent anti-viral properties.

Lung 10, LI 11, Stomach 44, Ren 22

Many of these herbs have been documented in scientific studies as useful to combat the common cold. The most promising appears to be Andrographis, which has studies that document its efficacy.[174,175] Echinacea is perhaps the most controversial herb in treating the cold. There are several meta studies on Echinacea that show that it is helpful in the treatment of colds and flus, and, it seems, an equal number that prove that it has no effect. More standardization is needed regarding the form and therapeutic dose before we can have clarity on the efficacy of this herb. From my conversations with more informed herbalists, the most potent phytochemical within Echinacea is Alkamides, which is not soluble in water and only presents in Echinacea Angustifolia roots and Echinacea Purpura flowers. Other herbs listed above have some scientific evidence but will require more intense scrutiny from the scientific community before they will become accepted as a valid treatment for the cold or flu.

Integrative Comments

Prior to my discovery of Second Brain-related colds, the use of Heat Toxin herbs was a primary part of my treatment for colds and flus as backed up by modern research. While I have developed a more comprehensive approach, these herbs deserve our attention and remain helpful for millions of Americans.[176] I do still prescribe these herbs from time to time, and it remains an effective treatment for many people who rely on these herbs as their sole treatment for their colds.

Damp and Summer Heat

A fourth category of heat is called Damp Heat, and is recognized by a combination of inflammation and mucous. A fifth heat category is Summer Heat, which is its own separate category, as seen below.

DAMPNESS

Dampness is a very useful concept in **TCM** that refers to symptoms involving mucus: post-nasal drip, runny nose or any other bodily mucus. Dampness is most easily seen as discharge associated with a cold such as a runny nose, post-nasal drip or the mucous associated with a productive cough. The innovation of the **TCM** concept of Dampness provides a means of treating a complex cold in a more complete way since herbs associated with dampness can often be combined with herbs that treat other aspects of a cold. The **TCM** pharmacopoeia includes many herbs that help reduce the production of mucus.

Symptoms associated with Dampness:

- Runny nose.
- Phlegmy cough.
- Post-nasal drip.
- Achiness, sluggishness, mental dullness.

Damp-Cold and Damp-Heat

Dampness is usually diagnosed with Heat or Cold patterns. The Damp-Cold Pattern simply means that discharge is clear or white without signs or symptoms of inflammation. The Damp-Heat Pattern means a patient does show signs and symptoms of inflammation such as yellowish, yellow or even green discharge from sinuses or a cough. Both types of dampness tend to be difficult to get rid of and Western medicine has few effective drugs to rid the body of excess mucus. By comparison, treating damp symptoms in **TCM** is relatively easy. Below is a list of the four common Damp and Damp-Heat colds and the typical herbs and acupressure/acupuncture points used to treat them.

Treatment of Damp-Heat

Cold Heat

SINUS INFECTION	LOOSE, PRODUCTIVE COUGH	POST-NASAL DRIP
Pen Men Kan Wan, including herbs such as Xanthum and Magnolia Flower	Er Chen Wan, including herbs such as Magnolia Bark, Mandarin Orange Peel, and Pinellia	Er Chen Wan, including herbs such as Aged Mandarin Orange Peel, Pinellia and Magnolia Bark
	Sp 9, Ren 12, Sp 6	

Heat Damp

SINUS INFECTION	LOOSE, PRODUCTIVE COUGH	POST-NASAL DRIP
Bi Yan Wan, including Scutellaria, Xanthium and Magnolia Flower	Huang Lian Wen Dan Tang, including Coptis, Scutellaria and Houttunia	Scutellaria Root, Coptis Root, Phellodendron Root
	Cold-Damp points plus St 44, LI 4, LU 5, Liv 2	

The **TCM** herbal formula used for Cold-Damp is primarily Er Chen WanTwo Peel decoction (aged, dried Mandarin orange and Poria) while the Damp-Heat formulas are Huang Lian Wen Dan Tang or Qing Qi Hua Tan. Refer to the herbal formula section for a full listing of herbs and dosages.

Summer Heat (exposure to Damp weather)

During my internship in China, I became sick within the first week of my three month stay, feeling constant fatigue and mental spaciness. I also suffered from a soft and loose stool, which I, for several weeks, mistook for mild food poisoning. During this time, I felt tired and mentally cloudy, and I dragged myself to classes and clinics while taking Wind-Heat herbal prescriptions. I finally received proper treatment from one of the highly-qualified teaching doctors in the outpatient clinic. His diagnosis: Summer Heat! Within hours of taking the Chinese herbs for Summer Heat, I had fully recovered. From this, I learned that Summer Heat is often overlooked by **TCM** practitioners. I also really misunderstood just how important proper diagnosis is in treating the common cold. I had tried several other **TCM** cold formulas with virtually no effect.

The primary symptom of Summer Heat is diarrhea or loose stool. Along with a loose stool, most people complain of whole-body achiness, fatigue and mental fog. Summer heat in **TCM** causes these symptoms due to a virus invading the large intestines.

The symptoms associated with Summer Heat are:

- Diarrhea or loose stool.
- Mild stomach cramps.
- Forehead banded headache.
- Lassitude.
- Ache throughout whole body.
- Chills.
- Absence of thirst.
- Nausea or queasiness.
- Aversion to greasy foods.
- Slippery pulse.
- Chills.
- Tongue is greasy with white or yellowish coating.

I treat a few patients each year with herbs and acupuncture for this condition. I can identify patients in the early stages of this cold, who only have a handful of the symptoms listed above. Research on this herbal formula is sparse, but a new research paper reviewing its efficacy on gastrointestinal problems has recently been published.[177] This comprehensive paper documents the anti-inflammatory and immune-stimulating characteristics of this formula and highlights that further research should be done to understand the effects of this herbal formula.

One helpful additional piece of information about Summer Heat is that there is rarely a sore throat or any sinus symptoms associated with it and frequently patients feel chilled. When you consider this category for yourself or your family, remember that this is essentially an intestinal flu so digestive symptoms are the key to getting this one right. Not everyone with this type of flu has diarrhea or even a loose stool, but may only have a very low appetite. It can look a lot like mild to moderate food poisoning, as many with food poisoning, have temporary diarrhea and feel quite sick, but the difference is Summer Heat colds last longer, sometimes a lot longer, than a bout of food poisoning which typically lasts no longer than 24 hours. The herbal and acupuncture/acupressure formulas for Summer Heat are both elegant and effective.

Treatment of Summer Heat

BODY ACHES, LOOSE STOOL, CHILLS	BODY ACHES, FRONTAL HEADACHE	BODY ACHES, LOOSE STOOL OR DIARRHEA, CHILLED, LOW APPETITE, FRONTAL PRESSURE HEADACHE
Huo Xiang Zheng Qi Tang, including herbs such as Pachouli, Magnolia Bark, Mandarin Orange Peel, Perilla Leaf	Pill Curing including herbs such as Poria, Chinese Barley, Pachouli, Gastrodia	Pachouli, Cardamon, Magnolia Bark *Common patent herbal formulas include Huo Xiang Zheng Qi Tang and Pill Curing*
UB 40, ST 25		UB 40, Sp 9 UB 58, ST 40

DRYNESS

Dryness refers to overexposure to a dry climate. Dryness Pattern is primarily used to treat patients with a dry cough, a dry throat and/or dry sinuses, and a tendency to be dehydrated or have damaged mucosal lining. Dryness is frequently associated with the end stage of a cold where all that remains is a dry cough and/or a feeling that the throat and sinuses are dry.

The symptoms are:

- Dry cough, no mucus.
- Dry mouth, lips.
- Dry throat.
- Dry sinuses.
- Increased thirst often unsatisfied by drinking water.

A person with Dryness symptoms has a dry, hacking cough and/or seemingly unending dry sinuses. Herbal treatments can provide rapid symptomatic relief. Below I provide a listing of common herbs and acupuncture/acupressure points used.

Treatment of Dryness

DRY COUGH	DRY SINUS
Sha Shen Mai Dong Tang, including herbs such as Raw Rehmannia, Glehnia, Ophiopogonis	Raw Rehmannia, Glehnia, Ophiopogonis, Xanthium
Ki 6, LU 7	

SUMMARY OF THE FIVE ENVIRONMENTAL PATTERNS

Together, these Five Environmental Patterns constitute a foundation in understanding the **TCM** approach to treating colds and flus. Each pattern has unique and different symptoms. While I no longer rely on this diagnostic system, I do find that it is helpful at times, and provides a foundation for understanding the importance of separating symptoms and tailoring treatments to match them.

There are only three additional causes of colds in **TCM** which should be included on this list to make it comprehensive: **Tai Yang** colds, Shao Yang colds and Chest Bi colds.

Three Additional TCM Patterns for Colds and Flu

The history of the development of **TCM** is long and interesting. The theoretical foundations of this fascinating medicine have evolved over time; doctors have formulated competing theories based on their clinical experience. A few of these innovations have survived the test of time. The main theory used to treat colds and flu is called the Five Environmental Patterns, summarized in the first part of this appendix. The primary competing theoretical framework for the treatment of colds and flu stems from a manuscript written by Zhang Zhongjing, a famous Second Century Chinese doctor. This doctor devised a different understanding of colds and flu based on experiments and innovations he discovered while working with patients during a flu pandemic that was ravaging the Chinese population at that time. The final section of this appendix explains two of the patterns that he formulated along with the herbal prescriptions that are used to treat them.

Two Cold Formulas from the *Shan Han Lun*

In this section, we will look at two of the most well-known herbal formulas created by Dr. Zhang Zhongjing as well as their theoretical foundation. Dr. Zhang Zhongjing's theory is outlined in a treatise called the *Shun Han Lun*, which translates to *Treatise On the Treatment of Acute Diseases Caused By Cold*. The theory created a competing diagnostic treatment framework of many diseases in **TCM**, including the common cold.

The two diagnoses and treatments are:

1. Tai Yang Cold/Flu (Tai is pronounced like "Tie," Yang -rhythms with "song").
2. Shao Yang Cold/Flu (pronounced like Shout without the "t" at the end).

Tai Yang and Shao Yang Cold or Flu

The *Shun Han Lun* was developed and codified by Zhang Zhongjing who wrote this classic seminal text in **TCM**, which is sometimes translated as the *Treatise On the Treatment of Acute Diseases Caused By Cold*. This important treatise was written sometime around 220 AD, which sheds light in a different way on the diagnosis and treatment of colds. This diagnostic method looks at disease in how they affect pairs of meridians. **Tai Yang** disorders, for instance, refer to the UB and SI meridians.

UB Meridian and SI Meridians are energy lines in the body that are used in the Six Stages. Together, they form the "**Tai Yang** Meridians".

Shao Yang disorders refer to the GB and SJ Meridians, which like the **Tai Yang** meridians, are paired together.

While there are four more pairings or meridians, we will focus only on **Tai Yang** and Shao Yang disorders as they are by far the most common pairings associated with the common cold. *The Shun Han Lun* was written in response to a flu epidemic in China during Zhang Zhongjing's time. He was among hundreds of Chinese doctors that were trying to find an effective method to treat the many desperately ill patients who were not responding to the more conventional standard of care.

During this epidemic, Dr. Zhang Zhongjing developed and wrote about a more effective treatment. The impact of this method stands as a pillar within **TCM** and he remains acknowledged as one of the most important and certainly famous of all practitioners through all the many centuries of **TCM**. Today, his treatise of *The Shun Han Lun* is still taught in advanced courses in Chinese medical schools, and he remains regarded as one of the founding fathers of **TCM**. The hospital in China where I did my internship had a large statue of Zhang Zhongjing in the entry plaza of the hospital.

Tai Yang/Stiff Neck Colds

Tai Yang colds are catalogued not so much by a fixed constellation of symptoms, like the environment factor colds in the previous section, but are more focused on the body and muscle tension that accompanies the cold symptoms. These muscular symptoms are not as obvious as the standard cold symptoms such as sore throat, fever or sinus congestion. For someone who is used to using palpation to search for painful tight muscles, such as an acupuncturist or massage therapist, this muscular tension can be quite obvious and easily revealed in a patient who may be otherwise unaware of underlying tension and pain.

Dr. Zhang Zhongjing discovered that colds and flus create lines of tension in the body that are consistent with particular types of colds. The **Tai Yang** cold, for instance, was found to create tension in the **Tai Yang** meridians. Today, using modern medical terminology, we would say that this tension was based on **Low Vagal Tone**, shunting **Acetylcholine** from the Vagus Nerve and thereby creating tension along the paraspinal muscles in the back and neck.

Dr. Zang then, using this as a theoretical framework, developed herbal formulas designed to relax muscles along the **Tai Yang** meridians and reduce pain throughout this part of the body, along with prescribing herbs to inhibit viruses (heat toxins). These formulations can still be found today in **TCM** dispensaries and acupuncture clinics, and stand as viable options against other herbal cold formulas. In the early days of my practice, I used these formulas often as they would help lessen symptoms in more severe colds and flus.

Every cold, regardless of its cause, whether from Wind Heat or Summer Heat, can be mild to miserable. **Tai Yang** colds are typically more severe than most colds or flus, especially if a high fever or chills develop. Here is a comprehensive list of the **Tai Yang** set of symptoms.

- Tight neck.
- Sinus congestion.
- Sore throat.
- Fatigue.
- Restlessness and a vague irritability.
- Chills/fever.
- Frontal headaches.
- Pulse is floating and tight.
- In advanced stages of the cold, a spasmodic cough is also present.

It is amazing that this diagnostic system, conceived in the 2nd century, is still used today. His innovations during that time reshaped Chinese Medicine and helped this diverse medical system become more effective in treating colds and flus. My premise that **Enteric Nervous System** viral colds cause temporary **Silent Reflux** symptoms was first envisioned because of this diagnostic system. The saying, "We stand on the shoulders of those who came before us" is good to remember. For this brilliant Chinese doctor, Zhang Zhongjing, who discovered this diagnosis, guided me to make further discoveries.

Treatment of Tai Yang Colds

SORE THROAT, STIFF NECK, SINUS CONGESTION	SORE THROAT, STIFF NECK, SINUS CONGESTION PLUS CHILLS
Chai Ge Jie Ji Tang, including herbs such as Bupleurum, Kudzu Root, Notopterygium Root	Mitake, Shitake, Chaga Mushrooms and other medicinal mushrooms
SI 4, UB 64, UB 57, UB10-12	

Integrative comments

A **Tai Yang** cold can respond favorably to a deep, long massage or acupuncture. The treatment should focus along the UB meridian along the cervical spine and the calf muscles. While this can be a very painful experience, the results can often take a lot of the misery out of a miserable cold. Acupuncture is far less painful and can be equally helpful, however. Placing needles in the UB 57 and 58 zone can provide an alternative method to treat **Tai Yang** colds.

Shao Yang Cold or Flu

Dr. Zhang Zhongjing, also developed a theory around a second meridian pairing called Shao Yang. Shao Yang has to do with a **Tai Yang** cold that is entering into a deeper layer of the muscle and body. Instead of the Cold Pattern entering the meridians in the back of the body (the **Tai Yang** meridians), the Shao Yang colds enter the meridians that traverse the sides of the body. The symptoms experienced with this type of cold tend to alternate between opposing symptoms such as fever and chills. Ironically, the Shao Yang patient tends to be more functional than the **Tai Yang** cold sufferer. The clinical picture resembles a stressed out student that has just completed a week of finals at school or the jet-lagged traveler that is "wired and tired" and can't seem to get meaningful rest or sleep.

Shao Yang colds symptoms include three or more of the following:

- Alternating chills and fever.
- Feeling stress similar to jet-lag.
- Variable symptoms.
- Fullness in the ribs and side rib regions.
- Mental restlessness.
- Bitter taste.
- Dry throat.
- Blurry vision.
- Bowstring pulse, in TCM this is a pounding pulse indicating the body is under stress.

The focus of the symptoms of the Shao Yang cold, like the **Tai Yang** cold are more on the physical body than on symptoms we typically associate with a head or chest cold. Symptoms such as fullness in the ribs, feeling stressed and mental restlessness seem weirdly out of place when we talk about cold symptoms.

Integrative Comments

I no longer use this approach when treating a cold, although I have seen it work. My approach now is exclusively on **ENS** viral colds and treating **Low Vagal Tone** as this approach works on releasing stress and restoring functional balance to the body on a deeper level by restoring the function of the **Parasympathetic Nervous System**.

Treatment of Shao Yang Colds

SHAO YANG COLD
Xiao Chai Hu Tang[178]
Including herbs such as Bupleurum, Scutellaria, Pinellia, Licorice *These herbs are ones included in Xiao Chai Hu Tang.*
Liver 3, Gall Bladder 44, Liver 14

Chest Bi Colds

Chest Bi colds are colds that are characterized by tightness in the chest, often causing difficulty and sometimes pain in breathing. This kind of cold is common to those who are prone to asthma. There are two types of Chest Bi colds. Cold Chest Bi and Chest Bi with heat.

Symptoms:

- Tight chest.
- Difficulty breathing or perhaps just difficulty taking a deep breath.
- Can have a wet or dry cough.
- Bowstring pulse.

Treatment of Chest Bi Colds

CHEST BI COLD
Gua Luo Zhi Shi Tang[179]
Trichosanthes Fruit, Fritillariae Cirrhosae Bulb, Aged Tangerine Peel, Balloon Flower Root, Aucklandiae Root, Amomi Fruit Sha, Cocos Mushroom, Gardenia Seed, Skullcap Root, Chinese Angelica Root, Licorice Root, Fresh Ginger Root, Bamboo Sap
Pericardium 6, Kidney 6, Lung 7, Spleen 4

Integrative Comments

This diagnosis and herbal formulation demonstrates the versatility and breadth of Chinese Medicine. I occasionally use this approach for patients with mild pneumonia or asthma symptoms that accompany a cold.

REFERENCES

1. Mäkelä MJ, Puhakka T, Ruuskanen O, et al. Viruses and bacteria in the etiology of the common cold. J Clin Microbiol. 1998;36(2):539–542.

2. Bischoff WE, Reid T, Russell GB, Peters TR. Transocular entry of seasonal influenza-attenuated virus aerosols and the efficacy of n95 respirators, surgical masks, and eye protection in humans. J Infect Dis. 2011 Jul 15; 204(2):193-9. PMID: 21673029.

3. Nocchi, S., et al. "In vitro cytotoxicity and anti-Herpes simplex virus type 1 activity of hydroethanolic extract, fractions, and isolated compounds from stem bark of Schinus terebinthifolius Raddi." Pharmacogn. Mag. 2016 Apr-Jun; 12(46): 160-4.

4. Simons, J., et al. "Succulent-type as sources of plant virus inhibitors." Phytopathology. 1963; 53: 677-83.

5. Prasertkul M, Puthavathana P, Sangsiriwut K, et al. Influenza A H5N1 replication sites in humans. Emerg Infect Dis. 2005;11(7):1036–1041. doi:10.3201/eid1107.041313.

6. Hamming, I.; Timens, W.; Bulthuis, M. L. C.; Lely, A. T.; Navis, G. J.; Goor, H. van (2004). "Tissue distribution of ACE2 protein, the functional receptor for SARS coronavirus. A first step in understanding SARS pathogenesis". The Journal of Pathology. 203 (2): 631–637. doi:10.1002/path.1570.

7. Ungaro RC, et al "What should gastroenterologists and patients know about COVID-19?" Clin Gastroenterol Hepatol 2020; Published March 17, 2020.

8. Gershon MD. The enteric nervous system: a second brain. Hosp Pract (1995). 1999;34(7):. doi:10.3810/hp.1999.07.153.

9. Gershon MD. Enteric serotonergic neurones ... finally!. J Physiol. 2009;587(3):507. doi:10.1113/jphysiol.2008.167676.

10. Gershon MD. 5-Hydroxytryptamine (serotonin) in the gastrointestinal tract. Curr Opin Endocrinol Diabetes Obes. 2013;20(1):14–21. doi:10.1097/MED.0b013e32835bc703.

11. Gershon MD, Tack J. The serotonin signaling system: from basic understanding to drug development for functional GI disorders. Gastroenterology. 2007;132(1):397–414. doi:10.1053/j.gastro.2006.11.002.

12. Terry N, Margolis KG. Serotonergic Mechanisms Regulating the GI Tract: Experimental Evidence and Therapeutic Relevance. Handb Exp Pharmacol. 2017;239:319–342. doi:10.1007/164_2016_103.

13. Gaude GS. Pulmonary manifestations of gastroesophageal reflux disease. Ann Thorac Med. 2009;4(3):115–123. doi:10.4103/1817-1737.53347.

14. Lee AS, Lee JS, He Z, Ryu JH. Reflux-Aspiration in Chronic Lung Disease. Ann Am Thorac Soc. 2020;17(2):155–164. doi:10.1513/AnnalsATS.201906-427CME.

15. Kellogg DL, Zhao JL, Coey U, Green JV (February 2005). "Acetylcholine-induced vasodilation is mediated by nitric oxide and prostaglandins in human skin". J. Appl. Physiol. 98 (2): 629–32. doi:10.1152/japplphysiol.00728.2004.

16. Kodama Y, Iino S, Shigemasa Y, Suzuki H. Properties of acetylcholine-induced relaxation of smooth muscle isolated from the proximal colon of the guinea-pig. J Smooth Muscle Res. 2010;46(4):185–200. doi:10.1540/jsmr.46.185.

17. Furchgott RF, Zawadzki JV. The obligatory role of endothelial cells in the relaxation of arterial smooth muscle by acetylcholine. Nature. 1980;288(5789):373–376. doi:10.1038/288373a0.

18. Zijlstra FJ, van den Berg-de Lange I, Huygen FJ, Klein J. Anti-inflammatory actions of acupuncture. Mediators Inflamm. 2003;12(2):59–69. doi:10.1080/0962935031000114943.

19. Kavoussi B, Ross BE. The neuroimmune basis of anti-inflammatory acupuncture. Integr Cancer Ther. 2007;6(3):251–257. doi:10.1177/1534735407305892.

20. McDonald JL, Cripps AW, Smith PK, Smith CA, Xue CC, Golianu B. The anti-inflammatory effects of acupuncture and their relevance to allergic rhinitis: a narrative review and proposed model. Evid Based Complement Alternat Med. 2013;2013:591796. doi:10.1155/2013/591796.

21. Pearce JMS. Silas Weir Mitchell (1829–1914) and causalgia. J Neurol Neurosurg Psychiatry 1990;53:763.

22. Drinking plenty of fluids may be harmful , Published: 26 February 2004; BMJ 328 doi:10.1136/bmj.328.7438.0-.

23. https://askabiologist.asu.edu/memory-b-cell.

24. See Hijacked: Our System is being hijacked by a Virusr for details on the viral cloning process.

25. We will learn more about the cleanup process in the EliminatingYour Cough by Clearing Out Clutter.

26. For more information on this process, refer to theWe will learn more about the cleanup process in the EliminatingYour Cough by Clearing Out Clutter h and Let the Acetylcholine flow: How to Open up blood and nerve flow to heal a Sinus Infection chapters.

27. NK cell development, homeostasis and function: parallels with CD8+ T cells. Joseph C. Sun & Lewis L. Lanier Nature Reviews Immunology volume 11, pages 645–657 (2011).

28. Streltsova MA, Erokhina SA, Kanevskiy LM, Lee DA, Telford WG, Sapozhnikov AM, et al. (2018) Analysis of NK cell clones obtained using interleukin-2 and gene-modified K562 cells revealed the ability of "senescent" NK cells to lose CD57 expression and start expressing NKG2A. PLoS ONE 13(12): e0208469. https://doi.org/10.1371/journal.pone.0208469.

29. Wachtel-Galor S, Szeto YT, Tomlinson B, et al: Ganoderma lucidum ('Lingzhi'): Acute and short-term biomarker response to supplementation. Int J Food Sci Nutr 55:75-83, 2004.

30. Guggenheim AG, Wright KM, Zwickey HL. Immune Modulation From Five Major Mushrooms: Application to Integrative Oncology. Integr Med (Encinitas). 2014;13(1):32-44.

31. Coutinho AE, Chapman KE. The anti-inflammatory and immunosuppressive effects of glucocorticoids, recent developments and mechanistic insights. Mol Cell Endocrinol. 2011;335(1):2–13. doi:10.1016/j.mce.2010.04.005.

32. Version:0.9 StartHTML:00000162 EndHTML:00000232 StartFragment:00000196 EndFragment:00000196 SourceURL:https://www.ncbi.nlm.nih.gov/pmc/articles/PMC3047790/.

33. Tetel MJ, de Vries GJ, Melcangi RC, Panzica G, O'Mahony SM. Steroids, stress and the gut microbiome-brain axis. J Neuroendocrinol. 2018;30(2):10.1111/jne.12548. doi:10.1111/jne.12548.

34. Coskun M. Intestinal epithelium in inflammatory bowel disease. Front Med (Lausanne). 2014;1:24. Published 2014 Aug 25. doi:10.3389/fmed.2014.00024.

35. ACUPUNCTURE FOR LOW BACK PAIN Manheimer E, White A, Berman B,et al. Ann Intern Med 2005;142:651–63.

36. Acupuncture for Chronic Pain: Update of an Individual Patient Data Meta-Analysis, Vickers, Andrew J. et al., The Journal of Pain, Volume 19, Issue 5, 455 - 474.

37. https://www.acponline.org/acp-newsroom/american-college-of-physicians-issues-guideline-for-treating-nonradicular-low-back-pain.

38. Haller H, Lauche R, Cramer H, et al. Craniosacral Therapy for the Treatment of Chronic Neck Pain: A Randomized Sham-controlled Trial. Clin J Pain. 2016;32(5):441-449. doi:10.1097/AJP.0000000000000290.

39. Hauser, W. E., Remington, J. S.: Effect of antibiotics on the immune response. Am. J. Med. 72 (1982) 711-716.

40. Rusznicwski, P & Soufflet, Christine & Barthélémy, P. (2008). Nonsteroidal anti-inflammatory drug use as a risk factor for gastro-oesophageal reflux disease: An observational study. Alimentary pharmacology & therapeutics. 28. 1134-9. 10.1111/j.1365-2036.2008.03821.x.

41. Denzler K, Moore J, Harrington H, et al. Characterization of the Physiological Response following In Vivo Administration of Astragalus membranaceus. Evid Based Complement Alternate Med. 2016;2016:6861078. doi:10.1155/2016/6861078.

42. Chong PP, Chin VK, Looi CY, Wong WF, Madhavan P, Yong VC. The Microbiome and Irritable Bowel Syndrome - A Review on the Pathophysiology, Current Research and Future Therapy [published correction appears in Front Microbiol. 2019 Aug 13;10:1870]. Front Microbiol. 2019;10:1136. Published 2019 Jun 10. doi:10.3389/fmicb.2019.01136.

43. Luo A, Leach ST, Barres R, Hesson LB, Grimm MC, Simar D. The Microbiota and Epigenetic Regulation of T Helper 17/Regulatory T Cells: In Search of a Balanced Immune System. Front Immunol. 2017;8:417. Published 2017 Apr 10. doi:10.3389/fimmu.2017.00417.

44. Lee YK, Menezes JS, Umesaki Y, Mazmanian SK. Proinflammatory T-cell responses to gut microbiota promote experimental autoimmune encephalomyelitis. Proc Natl Acad Sci U S A. 2011;108 Suppl 1(Suppl 1):4615–4622. doi:10.1073/pnas.1000082107.

45. Mori G, D'Amelio P, Faccio R, Brunetti G. The Interplay between the bone and the immune system. Clin Dev Immunol. 2013;2013:720504.

46. Ibid.

47. Jayaraj R, Megha P, Sreedev P. Organochlorine pesticides, their toxic effects on living organisms and their fate in the environment. Interdiscip Toxicol. 2016;9(3-4):90–100. doi:10.1515/intox-2016-0012.

48. Rainer H. Straub, The Complex Role of Estrogens in Inflammation, Endocrine Reviews, Volume 28, Issue 5, 1 August 2007, Pages 521–574, https://doi.org/10.1210/er.2007-0001

49. Margues M, et al. Low levels of 3,3'-diindolylmethane activate estrogen receptor alpha and induce proliferation of breast cancer cells in the absence of estradiol.BMC Cancer.2014 Jul 21;14:524.

50. https://www.epa.gov/fish-tech/epa-fda-advice-about-eating-fish-and-shellfish.

51. https://www.disabled-world.com/calculators-charts/fish-mercury.php.

52. Determination of MeHg in Environmental Sample Matrices Using Hg–Thiourea Complex Ion Chromatography with On-line Cold Vapor Generation and Atomic Fluorescence Spectrometric Detection Christopher W. Shade* and Robert J. M. Hudson Environmental Science & Technology 2005 39 (13), 4974-4982.

53. Kim KM, Kwon YG, Chung HT, et al. Methanol extract of Cordyceps pruinosa inhibits in vitro and in vivo inflammatory mediators by suppressing NF-κB activation. Toxicol Appl Pharmacol. 2003;190(1):1–8.

54. Takimoto H, Kato H, Kaneko M, Kumazawa Y. Amelioration of skewed Th1/ Th2 balance in tumor-bearing and asthma-induced mice by oral administration of Agaricus blazei extracts. Immunopharmacol Immunotoxicol. 2008;30(4):747–760.

55. Lin JG, Fan MJ, Tang NY, et al. An extract of Agaricus blazei Murill administered orally promotes immune responses in murine leukemia BALB/c mice in vivo. Integr Cancer Ther. 2012;11(1):29–36.

56. Gao Y, Tang W, Gao H, et al. Antimicrobial activity of the medicinal mushroom Ganoderma. Food Rev Int. 2005;21(2):211–229.

57. Gao Y, Zhou S, Jiang W, Huang M, Dai X. Effects of ganopoly (a Ganoderma lucidum polysaccharide extract) on the immune functions in advanced-stage cancer patients. Immunol Invest. 2003;32(3):201–215.

58. Zhang S, Nie S, Huang D, Li W, Xie M. Immunomodulatory effect of Ganoderma atrum polysaccharide on CT26 tumor-bearing mice. Food Chem. 2013;136(3–4):1213–1219.

59. Wang G, Zhao J, Liu J, Huang Y, Zhong JJ, Tang W. Enhancement of IL-2 and IFN-gamma expression and NK cells activity involved in the anti-tumor effect of ganoderic acid Me in vivo. Int Immunopharmacol. 2007;7(6):864–870.

60. Yue GG, Fung KP, Leung PC, Lau CB. Comparative studies on the immunomodulatory and antitumor activities of the different parts of fruiting body of Ganoderma lucidum and Ganoderma spores. Phytother Res. 2008;22(10):1282–1291.

61. Deng G, Lin H, Seidman A, et al. A phase I/II trial of a polysaccharide extract from Grifola frondosa (Maitake mushroom) in breast cancer patients: immunological effects. J Cancer Res Clin Oncol. 2009;135(9):1215–1221.

62. Kodama N, Harada N, Nanba H. A polysaccharide, extract from Grifola frondosa, induces Th-1 dominant responses in carcinoma-bearing BALB/c mice. Jpn J Pharmacol. 2002;90(4):357–360.

63. Masuda Y, Inoue M, Miyata A, Mizuno S, Nanba H. Maitake β-glucan enhances therapeutic effect and reduces myelosupression and nephrotoxicity of cisplatin in mice. Int Immunopharmacol. 2009;9(5):620–626.

64. Masuda Y, Murata Y, Hayashi M, Nanba H. Inhibitory effect of MD-Fraction on tumor metastasis: involvement of NK cell activation and suppression of intercellular adhesion molecule (ICAM)-1 expression in lung vascular endothelial cells. Biol Pharm Bull. 2008;31(6):1104–1108.

65. Inoue A, Kodama N, Nanba H. Effect of maitake (Grifola frondosa) D-fraction on the control of the T lymph node Th-1/Th-2 proportion. Biol Pharm Bull. 2002;25(4):536–540.

66. Kodama N, Mizuno S, Nanba H, Saito N. Potential antitumor activity of a low-molecular-weight protein fraction from Grifola frondosa through enhancement of cytokine production. J Med Food. 2010;13(1):20–30.

67. Harada N, Kodama N, Nanba H. Relationship between dendritic cells and the D-fraction-induced Th-1 dominant response in BALB/c tumor-bearing mice. Cancer Lett. 2003;192(2):181–187.

68. Svagelj M, Berovic M, Boh B, Menard A, Simcic S, Wraber B. Solid-state cultivation of Grifola frondosa (Dicks: Fr) S.F. Gray biomass and immunostimulatory effects of fungal intra- and extracellular beta-polysaccharides. N Biotechnol. 2008;25(2–3):150–156.

69. Lu H, Yang Y, Gad E, et al. Polysaccharide krestin is a novel TLR2 agonist that mediates inhibition of tumor growth via stimulation of CD8 T cells and NK cells. Clin Cancer Res. 2011;17(1):67–76.

70. Lu H, Yang Y, Gad E, et al. TLR2 agonist PSK activates human NK cells and enhances the antitumor effect of HER2-targeted monoclonal antibody therapy. Clin Cancer Res. 2011;17(21):6742–6753.

71. Lu H, Yang Y, Gad E, et al. Polysaccharide krestin is a novel TLR2 agonist that mediates inhibition of tumor growth via stimulation of CD8 T cells and NK cells. Clin Cancer Res. 2011;17(1):67–76.

72. Lin JG, Fan MJ, Tang NY, et al. An extract of Agaricus blazei Murill administered orally promotes immune responses in murine leukemia BALB/c mice in vivo. Integr Cancer Ther. 2012;11(1):29–36.

73. Gao Y, Zhou S, Jiang W, Huang M, Dai X. Effects of ganopoly (a Ganoderma lucidum polysaccharide extract) on the immune functions in advanced-stage cancer patients. Immunol Invest. 2003;32(3):201–215.

74. Wang G, Zhao J, Liu J, Huang Y, Zhong JJ, Tang W. Enhancement of IL-2 and IFN-gamma expression and NK cells activity involved in the anti-tumor effect of ganoderic acid Me in vivo. Int Immunopharmacol. 2007;7(6):864–870.

75. Wang PY, Zhu XL, Lin ZB. Antitumor and immunomodulatory effects of polysaccharides from broken-spore of Ganoderma lucidum. Front Pharmacol. 2012 Jul;3:135.

76. Chen WY, Yang WB, Wong CH, Shih DT. Effect of Reishi polysaccharides on human stem/progenitor cells. Bioorg Med Chem. 2010;18(24):8583–8591.

77. Masuda Y, Inoue H, Ohta H, Miyake A, Konishi M, Nanba H. Oral administration of soluble β-glucans extracted from Grifola frondosa induces systemic antitumor immune response and decreases immunosuppression in tumor-bearing mice. Int J Cancer. 2013;133(1):108–119.

78. Torkelson CJ, Sweet E, Martzen MR, et al. Phase 1 clinical trial of Trametes versicolor in women with breast cancer. ISRN Oncol. 2012;2012:251632.

79. Arata S, Watanabe J, Maeda M, et al. Continuous intake of the Chaga mushroom (Inonotus obliquus) aqueous extract suppresses cancer progression and maintains body temperature in mice. Heliyon. 2016;2(5):e00111. Published 2016 May 12. doi:10.1016/j.heliyon.2016.e00111.

80. Won DP, Lee JS, Kwon DS, Lee KE, Shin WC, Hong EK. Immunostimulating activity by polysaccharides isolated from fruiting body of Inonotus obliquus. Mol Cells. 2011;31(2):165–173. doi:10.1007/s10059-011-0022-x.

81. https://www.cochrane.org/CD006895/ARI_probiotics-live-micro-organisms-to-prevent-upper-respiratory-tract-infections-urtis-for-example-the-common-cold.

82. Hao Q, Dong BR, Wu T. Probiotics for preventing acute upper respiratory tract infections. Cochrane Database of SystematicReviews2015, Issue 2. Art. No.: CD006895. DOI: 10.1002/14651858.CD006895.pub3.

83. Minna K. Salminen, Soile Tynkkynen, Hilpi Rautelin, Maija Saxelin, Martti Vaara, Petri Ruutu, Seppo Sarna, Ville Valtonen, Asko Järvinen, Lactobacillus Bacteremia during a Rapid Increase in Probiotic Use of Lactobacillus rhamnosus GG in Finland, Clinical Infectious Diseases, Volume 35, Issue 10, 15 November 2002, Pages 1155–1160, https://doi.org/10.1086/342912.

84. Kumpu M, Kekkonen RA, Kautiainen H, et al. Milk containing probiotic lactobacillus rhamnosus GG and respiratory illness in children: A randomized, double-blind, placebo controlled trial. Eur J Clin Nutr. 2012;66(9):1020-1023.

85. Chen L, Xu A, Yin N, et al. Enhancement of immune cytokines and splenic CD4+ T cells by electroacupuncture at ST36 acupoint of SD rats. PLoS One. 2017;12(4):e0175568. Published 2017 Apr 13. doi:10.1371/journal.pone.0175568.

86. Johnston MF, Ortiz Sánchez E, Vujanovic NL, Li W. Acupuncture May Stimulate Anticancer Immunity via Activation of Natural Killer Cells. Evid Based Complement Alternat Med. 2011;2011:481625. doi:10.1093/ecam/nep236.

87. Takayama S, Watanabe M, Kusuyama H, et al. Evaluation of the effects of acupuncture on blood flow in humans with ultrasound color Doppler imaging. Evid Based Complement Alternat Med. 2012;2012:513638. doi:10.1155/2012/513638.

88. Prasad AS. Zinc in human health: effect of zinc on immune cells. Mol Med. 2008;14(5-6):353–357. doi:10.2119/2008-00033.Prasad.

89. Z Zakay-Rones et al. Randomized study of the efficacy and safety of oral elderberry extract in the treatment of influenza A and B virus infections. J Int Med Res 2004; 32:132.

90. Segerstrom SC, Miller GE. Psychological Stress and the Human Immune System: A Meta-Analytic Study of 30 Years of Inquiry. Psychological bulletin. 2004;130(4):601-630. doi:10.1037/0033-2909.130.4.601.

91. As described in the Second Brain Chapter.

92. Mayer EA. Gut feelings: the emerging biology of gut-brain communication. Nat Rev Neurosci. 2011;12(8):453–466. Published 2011 Jul 13. doi:10.1038/nrn3071.

93. See the Second Brain chapter for a more basic introduction to the ENS.

94. Milovanovic B, Filipovic B, Mutavdzin S, et al. Cardiac autonomic dysfunction in patients with gastroesophageal reflux disease. World J Gastroenterol. 2015;21(22):6982–6989. doi:10.3748/wjg.v21.i22.6982.

95. Spiller R, Lam C. An Update on Post-infectious Irritable Bowel Syndrome: Role of Genetics, Immune Activation, Serotonin and Altered Microbiome. J Neurogastroenterol Motil. 2012;18(3):258–268. doi:10.5056/jnm.2012.18.3.258.

96. udo N, Chida Y, Aiba Y, et al. Postnatal microbial colonization programs the hypothalamic-pituitary-adrenal system for stress response in mice. J Physiol. 2004;558(Pt 1):263–275. doi:10.1113/jphysiol.2004.063388.

97. Ibid.

98. Liu RT. The microbiome as a novel paradigm in studying stress and mental health. Am Psychol. 2017;72(7):655–667. doi:10.1037/amp0000058.

99. Hart AL, Al-Hassi HO, Rigby RJ, et al. Characteristics of intesti-nal dendritic cells in inflammatory bowel diseases.Gastroenterology. 2005;129(1):50-65.

100. See the Shots Fired Chapter for more specific information on Macrophages.

101. Gareau, MG, Silva, MA, and Perdue, MH (2008). Pathophysiological mechanisms of stress-induced intestinal damage. Curr Mol Med. 8, 274-281.

102. Dinan TG, Cryan JF. Melancholic microbes: a link between gut microbiota and depression? Neurogastroenterol Motil 2013; 25: 713–719.

103. Cryan JF, O'Mahony SM. The microbiome-gut-brain axis: from bowel to behavior. Neurogastroenterol Motil 2011; 23: 187–192.

104. Rogers, G.B., Keating, D., Young, R.P., Wong, M.T., Licinio, J., & Wesselingh, S.L. (2016). From gut dysbiosis to altered brain function and mental illness: mechanisms and pathways. Molecular Psychiatry.

105. Gershon MD. 5-Hydroxytryptamine (serotonin) in the gastrointestinal tract. Current opinion in endocrinology, diabetes, and obesity. 2013;20(1):14-21. doi:10.1097/MED.0b013e32835bc703.

106. Krueger PM, Friedman EM. Sleep Duration in the United States: A Cross-sectional Population-based Study. American Journal of Epidemiology. 2009;169(9):1052-1063. doi:10.1093/aje/kwp023.

107. Werner GG, Ford BQ, Mauss IB, Schabus M, Blechert J, Wilhelm FH. High cardiac vagal control is related to better subjective and objective sleep quality. Biol Psychol. 2015;106:79–85. doi:10.1016/j.biopsycho.2015.02.004.

108. Prather AA, Vogelzangs N, Penninx BWJH. Sleep duration, insomnia, and markers of systemic inflammation: Results from the Netherlands Study of Depression and Anxiety (NESDA). Journal of psychiatric research. 2015;60:95-102. doi:10.1016/j.jpsychires.2014.09.018.

109. Cohen S, Doyle WJ, Alper CM, Janicki-Deverts D, Turner RB. Sleep Habits and Susceptibility to the Common Cold. Archives of internal medicine. 2009;169(1):62-67. doi:10.1001/archinternmed.2008.505.

110. Tetel, M.J., Vries, G.J., Melcangi, R.C., Panzica, G., & O'Mahony, S.M. (2018). Steroids, stress and the gut microbiome-brain axis. Journal of neuroendocrinology, 30 2.

111. Karen Lee Ann Chen, Xiaoji Liu, Yiru Chen Zhao, Kadriye Hieronymi, Gianluigi Rossi, Loretta Sue Auvil, Michael Welge, Colleen Bushell, Rebecca Lee Smith, Kathryn E. Carlson, Sung Hoon Kim, John A. Katzenellenbogen, Michael Joseph Miller, Zeynep Madak-Erdogan. Long-Term Administration of Conjugated Estrogen and Bazedoxifene Decreased Murine Fecal β-Glucuronidase Activity Without Impacting Overall Microbiome Community. Scientific Reports, 2018; 8 (1) DOI: 10.1038/s41598-018-26506-1.

112. Cindy Pensec, Dominique Guenot, Loreley Calvet, Caroline Mignard, Olivier Duchamp, Thomas Carton, Sébastien Leuillet, Hervé M. Blottière and Françoise Le Vacon, Cancer Res July 1 2019 (79) (13 Supplement) 662; DOI: 10.1158/1538-7445.AM2019-662.

113. Dudek-Wicher RK, Junka A, Bartoszewicz M. The influence of antibiotics and dietary components on gut microbiota. Prz Gastroenterol. 2018;13(2):85-92.

114. James, D. V. B., Munson, S. C., Maldonado-Martin, S., & Croix, M. B. A. D. S. (2012). Heart rate variability: Effect of exercise intensity on postexercise response. Research Quarterly for Exercise and Sport, 83(4), 533-9.

115. See the Shots Fired Chapter for details on the Innate Immune Response.

116. Mishra LC, Singh BB, Dagenais S. Scientific basis for the therapeutic use of Withania somnifera (ashwagandha): a review. Altern Med Rev. 2000;5(4):334-346.

117. Kuo J, Chen KW, Cheng IS, et al. The effect of eight weeks of supplementation with Eleutherococcus senticosus on endurance capacity and metabolism in human. Chin J Physiol.2010 Apr 30;53(2):105-11.

118. Olsson EM, von Scheele B, Panossian AG. A randomised, double-blind, placebo-controlled, parallel-group study of the standardised extract shr-5 of the roots of Rhodiola rosea in the treatment of subjects with stress-related fatigue. Planta Med. Feb 2009;75(2):105-112.

119. https://www.health.harvard.edu/blog/new-survey-reveals-the-rapid-rise-of-yoga-and-why-some-people-still-havent-tried-it-201603079179.

120. Yoga Journal and Yoga Alliance: 2016 Yoga in America Study. Yoga Journal, May 11, 2016. https://www.yogaalliance.org/Portals/0/2016 Yoga in America Study RESULTS.pdf.

121. A systematic review of randomised control trials on the effects of yoga on stress measures and mood. Pascoe, Michaela C. et al. Journal of Psychiatric Research , Volume 68 , 270 - 282.

122. N. Hartfiel, C. Burton, J. Rycroft-Malone, G. Clarke, J. Havenhand, S. B. Khalsa, R. T. Edwards; Yoga for reducing perceived stress and back pain at work, Occupational Medicine, Volume 62, Issue 8, 1 December 2012, Pages 606–612, https://doi.org/10.1093/occmed/kqs168.

123. Oke SL, Tracey KJ. The inflammatory reflex and the role of complementary and alternative medical therapies. Ann N Y Acad Sci. 2009;1172:172–180. doi:10.1196/annals.1393.013.

124. Ladan Eshkevari, Susan E. Mulroney, Rupert Egan, Lixing Lao; Effects of Acupuncture, RU-486 on the Hypothalamic-Pituitary-Adrenal Axis in Chronically Stressed Adult Male Rats, Endocrinology, Volume 156, Issue 10, 1 October 2015, Pages 3649–3660, https://doi.org/10.1210/EN.2015-1018.

125. Jerath R., Edry J.W., Barnes V.A., Jerath V. Physiology of long pranayamic breathing: neural respiratory elements may provide a mechanism that explains how slow deep breathing shifts the autonomic nervous system. Med Hypotheses, 2006; 67(3), 566-571.

126. do Prado, A., et al. "Schinus molle essential oil as a potential source of bioactive compounds: antifungal and antibacterial properties." J. Appl. Microbiol. 2019 Feb; 126(2): 516-522.Arpini, C., et al. "Purpuriocillium lilacinum infection in captive loggerhead sea turtle hatchlings. Med. Mycol. Case Rep. 2018 Oct 25;23:8-11.

127. Ennigrou, A., et al. "Assessing the fatty acid, essential oil composition, their radical scavenging and antibacterial activities of Schinus terebinthifolius Raddi leaves and twigs." J. Food Sci. Technol. 2018 Apr; 55(4): 1582-1590.

128. Scheid, T., et al. "Effects of Methanol fraction from leaves of Schinus terebinthifolius Raddi on nociception and spinal-cord oxidative biomarkers in Rats with neuropathic pain." Evid. Based Complement. Alternat. Med. 2018 May; 2018: 5783412.

129. Estevão, L., et al. "Schinus terebinthifolius Raddi (Aroeira) leaves oil attenuates inflammatory responses in cutaneous wound healing in mice." Acta Cir. Bras. 2017 Sep; 32(9): 726-735.

130. Nunes-Neto, P., et al. "The effect of Schinus terebinthifolius Raddi (Anacardiaceae) bark extract on histamine-induced paw edema and ileum smooth muscle contraction." Evid. Based Complement. Alternat. Med. 2017; 2017: 1416375.

131. Gaude GS. Pulmonary manifestations of gastroesophageal reflux disease. Ann Thorac Med. 2009;4(3):115–123. doi:10.4103/1817-1737.53347.

132. Ibid.

133. Zijlstra FJ, van den Berg-de Lange I, Huygen FJ, Klein J. Anti-inflammatory actions of acupuncture. Mediators Inflamm. 2003;12(2):59–69. doi:10.1080/0962935031000114943.

134. Park JY, Namgung U. Electroacupuncture therapy in inflammation regulation: current perspectives. J Inflamm Res. 2018;11:227–237. Published 2018 May 17. doi:10.2147/JIR.S141198.

135. Mori H, Nishijo K, Kawamura H, Abo T. Unique immunomodulation by electro-acupuncture in humans possibly via stimulation of the autonomic nervous system. Neurosci Lett. 2002;320(1-2):21–24. doi:10.1016/s0304-3940(02)00012-5.

136. McDonald JL, Cripps AW, Smith PK, Smith CA, Xue CC, Golianu B. The anti-inflammatory effects of acupuncture and their relevance to allergic rhinitis: a narrative review and proposed model. Evid Based Complement Alternat Med. 2013;2013:591796. doi:10.1155/2013/591796.

137. Jaggupilli A, et al. Analysis of the expression of human bitter taste receptors in extraoral tissues. Mol Cell Biochem. 2017 Feb;426(1-2):137-147.

138. Yu Y, et al. Berberine induces GLP-1 secretion through activation of bitter taste receptor pathways. Biochem Pharmacol. 2015 Sep 15;97(2):173-7.

139. McMullen MK, Whitehouse JM, Towell A. Bitters: Time for a New Paradigm. Evid Based Complement Alternat Med. 2015;2015:670504. doi:10.1155/2015/670504.

140. Gaude GS,. Op. Cit.

141. Ibid.

142. https://acpinternist.org/archives/2014/03/GERD.htm.

143. Gaude GS, Op Cit.

144. Ibid.

145. https://acpinternist.org/archives/2014/03/GERD.htm.

146. Madanick RD. Management of GERD-Related Chronic Cough. Gastroenterol Hepatol (N Y). 2013;9(5):311–313.

147. Weng H, Li JG, Mao Z, et al. Probiotics for Preventing Ventilator-Associated Pneumonia in Mechanically Ventilated Patients: A Meta-Analysis with Trial Sequential Analysis. Front Pharmacol. 2017;8:717. Published 2017 Oct 9. doi:10.3389/fphar.2017.00717.

148. Anon JB. Upper respiratory infections. Am J Med. 2010;123(4 Suppl):S16-S25. doi:10.1016/j.amjmed.2010.02.003.

149. See the Shots Fired Chapter for more details on this winding down of the Immune Response

150. Fiorucci S, Biagioli M, Zampella A, Distrutti E. Bile Acids Activated Receptors Regulate Innate Immunity. Front Immunol. 2018;9:1853. Published 2018 Aug 13. doi:10.3389/fimmu.2018.01853.

151. Lee RJ, Cohen NA. The emerging role of the bitter taste receptor T2R38 in upper respiratory infection and chronic rhinosinusitis. Am J Rhinol Allergy. 2013;27(4):283–286. doi:10.2500/ajra.2013.27.3911.

152. Head K, Chong LY, Piromchai P, et al. Systemic and topical antibiotics for chronic rhinosinusitis. Cochrane Database Syst Rev. 2016;4:CD011994. Published 2016 Apr 26. doi:10.1002/14651858.CD011994.pub2.

153. Pfab F, Schalock PC, Napadow V, Athanasiadis GI, Huss-Marp J, Ring J. Acupuncture for allergic disease therapy--the current state of evidence. Expert Rev Clin Immunol. 2014;10(7):831–841. doi:10.1586/1744666X.2014.924855.

154. Lee-Wong M, Karagic M, Doshi A, Gomez S, Resnick D. An osteopathic approach to chronic sinusitis. J Aller Ther. 2011;2(2): 109. doi:10.4172/2155-6121.1000109.

155. Severe Outcomes Among Patients with Coronavirus Disease 2019 (COVID-19) — United States, February 12–March 16, 2020. MMWR Morb Mortal Wkly Rep 2020;69:343-346. DOI: http://dx.doi.org/10.15585/mmwr.mm6912e2.

156. Ibid.

157. Ibid.

158. https://elifesciences.org/articles/16758.

159. https://www.cdc.gov/flu/pdf/freeresources/updated/antiviral-factsheet-updated.pdf.

160. Venkatesh, S. & Memish, Z.A. (2004). SARS: the new challenge to international health and travel medicine. EMHJ - Eastern Mediterranean Health Journal, 10 (4-5), 655-662, 2004.

161. WHO global report on traditional and complementary medicine 2019. Geneva: World Health Organization; 2019. Licence: CC BY-NC-SA 3.0 IGO.

162. https://www.ncbi.nlm.nih.gov/pmc/articles/PMC4728566/.

163. Quercetin and the Flu, American Journal of Physiology-Regulatory, Integrative and Comparative Physiology. J. Mark Davis, E.A. Murphy, J.L. McClellan, M.D. Carmichael, and J.D. Gangemi.

164. https://www.nih.gov/news-events/nih-research-matters/flu-virus-fortified-colder-weather.

165. https://outlandermedicine.com/2016/08/29/la-grippe-influenza-at-ardsmuir/.

166. Cardiovascular effects of ginger aqueous extract and its phenolic constituents are mediated through multiple pathways. Ghayur MN1, Gilani AH, Afridi MB, Houghton PJ. Vascul Pharmacol. 2005 Oct;43(4):234-41. Epub 2005 Sep 12.

167. Pharmacological studies on Chinese cinnamon. II. Effects of cinnamaldehyde on the cardiovascular and digestive systems. Harada M, Yano S. Chem Pharm Bull (Tokyo). 1975 May; 23(5):941-7.

168. Treatment of perennial allergic rhinitis using Shi-Bi-Lin, a Chinese herbal formula, Journal of ethnopharmacology 122(1):100-5 · February 2009 DOI: 10.1016/j.jep.2008.12.005.

169. Effect of a Chinese herbal formula, Shi-Bi-Lin, on an experimental model of allergic rhinitis. Zhao Y, van Hasselt CA, Woo JK, Chen GG, Wong YO, Wang LH, Leung PC. Ann Allergy Asthma Immunol. 2006 Jun;96(6):844-50.

170. Dharmananda S. Safety issues affecting Chinese herbs: The case of Xanthium. Institute for Traditional Medicine- European Branch 2003; 1:1-8.

171. Poivre M, Duez P. Biological activity and toxicity of the Chinese herb Magnolia officinalis Rehder & E. Wilson (Houpo) and its constituents. J Zhejiang Univ Sci B. 2017;18(3):194–214. doi:10.1631/jzus.B1600299.

172. Echinacea is not a TCM herb but is frequently categorized in this category by knowledgeable herbalist such as Michael and Leslie Tierra.

173. Usnea is another non TCM herb which I put in this category based on the work of Christopher Hobbs and the American Botanical Society as well as my own clinical experience.

174. Efficacy of Andrographis paniculata, Nees for pharyngotonsillitis in adults.

175. Thamlikitkul V1, Dechatiwongse T, Theerapong S, Chantrakul C, Boonroj P, Punkrut W, Ekpalakorn W, Boontaeng N, Taechaiya S, Petcharoen S, et al.

176. Coon J.T. and E. Ernst: Andrographis Paniculata in the Treatment of Upper Respiratory Tract Infections: A Systematic Review of Safety and Efficacy. Planta Med 2004.

177. Clarke TC, Black LI, Stussman BJ, Barnes PM, Nahin RL. Trends in the use of complementary health approaches among adults: United States, 2002–2012. National health statistics reports; no 79. Hyattsville, MD: National Center for Health Statistics. 2015.

178. Zhao M, Chen Y, Wang C, et al. Systems Pharmacology Dissection of Multi-Scale Mechanisms of Action of Huo-Xiang-Zheng-Qi Formula for the Treatment of Gastrointestinal Diseases. Front Pharmacol. 2019;9:1448. Published 2019 Jan 11. doi:10.3389/fphar.2018.01448.

179. Zheng N, Dai J, Cao H, et al. Current understanding on antihepatocarcinoma effects of xiao chai hu tang and its constituents. Evid Based Complement Alternat Med. 2013;2013:529458. doi:10.1155/2013/529458.

GLOSSARY

Acetylcholine – The main neurotransmitter released by the nervous system and the main neurotransmitter released by the Parasympathetic Nervous System to activate the "rest and digest" response.

Acetylcholine Shunt – A shunting or cutting off the supply of Acetylcholine to the surrounding muscles. This always causes muscle tension.

Acquired Immune Response – Part of the immune system that we acquire as we grow up. The Acquired Immune Response is a far more sophisticated and complex system that has a far more targeted response to pathogens.

Adaptation or Resistance Stage – The second phase of the stress response associated with ongoing stress. The main hormone associated with Cortisone.

Adaptive Humoral Response – The predominant part of the immune system that dominates the "humors" (an old medical term that refers to the interstitial fluids between the cells). The cell that provides the Adaptive Humoral Response is called the B-cell.

Adrenaline – The main hormone that dominates the Alarm Stage of the stress response. This ramps up the heart rate and energy in the body temporarily but can overtax our bodies if we activate this stress response too much.

Alarm Stage – The acute phase of stress associated with the release of adrenaline.

ANS – The Autonomic Nervous System

Assassin Army – T-cytotoxic cells and NK cells.

Autonomic Nervous System (ANS) – The part of the nervous system dedicated to the Stress Response.

B-cell – The cell that forms the Adaptive Humoral Response, which through various processes, helps to eliminate pathogens in the interstitial fluids.

B-cell Librarian Army – B-memory cells that carry a chemical memory of every virus strain you have ever caught.

B-cell Membrane-Bound Antibody – The part of a matching B-cell that binds to an MHC.

B-memory Cells – a B-cell that carries a chemical "memory" of the matching a virus or pathogen that we have had before. Presumably there are B-memory cells for every infection we've ever had.

Bile Salts – Chemicals produced by the liver that stimulate Vagal Tone.

CAM – Complementary and Alternative Medicine

Cell-Mediated Immune Response – This is an immune response controlled by T-cells that helps the body kill infected cells.

CNS – Central Nervous System. Also referred to as the brain.

Cortisol – The main hormone that dominates the Adaptation or Resistance Stage. This hormone helps keep your energy up but has many downsides for those who suffer from chronic stress.

Cytokines – Chemicals that stimulate the release of immune cells.

Cytotoxic T-cells – T-cells that kill virally-infected cells.

Dendritic Immune Cells – Innate immune cells that engulf pathogens and alert the acquired immune response associated with nerve tissue.

DNA – DNA provides the code for the cell's activities, while RNA converts that code into proteins to carry out cellular functions.

Dopamine – The hormone primarily associated with motivation.

ENS – Enteric Nervous System

ENS Viral Cold or Flu – The main site of a cold or flu viral infection. It means that the Enteric Nervous System becomes infected and initiates symptoms such as a fever, sore throat and a tight neck.

ENS Zone – The area above the navel and below the rib cage.

ENS/Epigastric Area – The area above the navel and below the rib cage.

Enteric Nervous System (ENS) – The network of nerves located in the gut that control digestion, produces 90% of the body's serotonin and 50% of the body's dopamine, and communicates information to the central nervous system.

Epigastric Area – The area above the navel and below the rib cage.

Estrogen – One of the key chemicals that help regulate menstruation.

Estrogen Dominance – An imbalance of estrogen and progesterone that causes PMS, hot flashes and other problems.

First Phase of a Cold – The first stage of a cold characterized by fever, a sore throat and fatigue.

GABA – A neurochemical associated with the parasympathetic nervous system.

GERD – Heartburn caused by inflammation of the lower esophageal sphincter.

Gut Brain Axis – The convergence of the Enteric Nervous System, the Gut Microbiome, the Autonomic Nervous System (including the Vagal Nerve) and the brain. This system has a profound effect on our digestion, mood and stress levels.

Gut Microbiome – The bacteria that forms the lining of the intestines. This bacterial lining helps with digestion, produces nutrients and sends messages to the brain via the enteric nervous system.

Humoral Immune Response – This is another term for the Adaptive Humoral Response.

Humors – The extracellular fluid.

Hypothalmus Pituitary Adrenal Axis (HPA) – The redundant part of the Alarm Stage of the stress response that activates adrenaline through the hypothalmus, pituitary and Adrenal glands.

Immune System – A general term for the system of white blood cells that fight infections in the body. This term also covers the skill that also protects us from infection.

Influenza A, Influenza B, and Influenza C – Viral strains of the flu (influenza).

Innate (or non-specific) Immune Response – Immune response's part of our first line of attack on viruses and other invaders. We say it is non-specific because it performs the same action regardless of the pathogen.

Irritable Bowel Syndrome – This is a common condition that means a person has chronic bowel problems such as diarrhea or constipation.

Leaky Gut – Increased intestinal permeability that causes bacteria (endotoxins) and other debris to leak through the intestinal walls into the interstitial fluid.

Low Vagal Tone – A condition where the nerve conduction and energy of the Vagus nerve is suppressed which results in a disabling of the Parasympathetic Nervous System Response, an exaggerated pro-inflammatory gut environment, and a suppression of the mucosal immune response.

Lower Esophageal Sphincter – The valve is located in the diaphragm where the stomach and esophagus meet that prevents the backflow of acid and food from backing up the esophagus.

Lymphocyte – A general term for an immune cell.

Macrophages – One of the main Innate Immune cells. Macrophages engulf pathogens and display MHCs. Sometimes referred to as the garbage collector of the body.

Major Histocompatibility Complex – When a macrophage or B-cell engulfs a virus or other pathogen, it displays fragments of this pathogen on its surface. This forms a surface receptor that is called a Major Histocompatibility Complex.

MHC – Major Histocompatibility Complex

Natural Killer Cell – Cytotoxic cells that are part of the innate immune response. These cells cannot clone themselves.

NK Cell – Natural Killer Cells

Novel Virus – A new viral strain which is the result of a viral mutation. This means s T-memory cells don't have a memory of this virus.

NSAIDS – Common over the counter painkillers/anti-inflammatories medications such as Ibuprofen and Motrin.

Organochlorines – Chemicals like those found in pesticides, herbicides, chlorine and pollution.

Organophosphates – Chemicals like those found in pesticides, herbicides, chlorine and pollution.

Osteoclasts – Cells within our bones that help the body destroy old bone so that it can replace it with new bone.

Parasympathetic Nervous System – The part of the Stress Response associated with the rest and digest stage of the stress response.

Pathogen – Any organism, such as bacteria or virus, that can cause disease.

Pro-Inflammatory Response – An immune response characterized by heightened inflammation, fever, redness and pain.

Proton Pump Inhibitors – Common medications used to treat GERD, which is commonly called heartburn.

Rhinovirus – The most common viral strain associated with the common cold.

RNA – DNA provides the code for the cell's activities, while RNA converts that code into proteins to carry out cellular functions.

Second Brain – The Enteric Nervous System.

Second Phase of a Cold – The second phase of a cold is characterized by a sinus or a chest cold. The second phase does not have fevers, chills or a significant sore throat associated with it.

Serotonin – The hormone associated with happiness.

Silent Reflux – A milder version of GERD causing intermittent symptoms such as waking with a sore throat or trouble swallowing.

Stress Response – The overarching term that refers to the Autonomic Nervous System and the HPA Axis.

Sympathetic Nervous System (SNS) – The part of the Stress Response associated with the Alarm stage of the stress response.

T- memory Cells – A T-memory cells that carry a chemical memory of every virus strain you have ever caught.

T-helper Cells – A T-cell that helps B-cells and T-Cytotoxic cells initiate and sustain the cloning process.

T-Regulatory Cells – A broad term that refers to cells that turn up the immune response like T-helper cells or ones that turn it down like **T-Regulatory** cells.

Tai Yang/ Stiff Neck Cold – A Chinese diagnosis for a cold or flu that has symptoms that include a stiff neck and fever and chills.

TCM – Traditional Chinese Medicine

Temporary Silent Reflux – A condition which means that a person temporarily develops Silent Reflux symptoms such as the onset of a cold or flu.

TH1 – A term that indicates the immune system is anti-inflammatory mode.

Th17 Cells – Th17 Cells are one of the activating chemicals that stimulate NK Cells. This means an unhealthy Gut Microbiome may inhibit the release of these vital Cytokines.

TH2 – A term that indicates the immune system is pro-inflammatory mode.

Top Down Stress Response – Stress associated with life challenges such as a job loss or divorce or money difficulties.

Traditional Chinese Medicine (TCM) – Holistic medical practices from China that include acupuncture, cupping, and moxa.

Trigeminal Nerve – A cranial nerve that exits out of the junction of the top of the neck and splits into three branches. One travels to the sinuses, one to the temporal area, and one to the mouth.

Vagus Nerve – A pair of cranial nerves that lead from the brainstem to the gut. This nerve serves as a communication link between the ENS and the brain and is the main branch of the Parasympathetic Nerve.

Viral Tissue Tropism – Cells or tissues that support the growth of a virus.

WBC – White Blood Cell

White Blood Cell – A general term for an immune cell.

WHO – World Health Organization

CPSIA information can be obtained
at www.ICGtesting.com
Printed in the USA
LVHW081318091020
668419LV00015B/951

9 781735 419619